LYME DISEASE

medical myopia and the hidden global epidemic

A Patient's Guide to Navigating the Labyrinth of Diagnosis and Treatment

Dr Bernard Raxlen

Contributions from Allie Cashel
(former patient & author of *Suffering the Silence*)
and tick-borne disease thought leaders from around the world

Dr Lambert • Dr Perronne • Dr Armstrong
• Dr McManus • Dr Alonso Canal • Dr Morales
• Dr Schwarzbach • Zhaneta Misho
• Dr Cook • Jenna Luché-Thayer
Illustrations and cover image by Rolo Ledesma

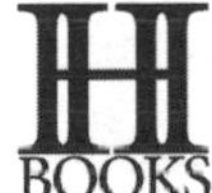

Hammersmith Health Books
London, UK

First published in 2019 by Hammersmith Health Books – an imprint of Hammersmith Books Limited
4/4A Bloomsbury Square, London WC1A 2RP, UK
www.hammersmithbooks.co.uk

Disclaimer: The information in this book is of a general nature and is meant for educational purposes only. It is not intended as medical advice. The contents may not be used to treat, or diagnose, any particular disease or any particular person. Applying elements from this publication does not constitute a professional relationship or professional advice or services. No endorsement or warranty is explicitly given or implied by any entity connected to this content.

As always, if you are have pre-existing health issues and especially if you are taking any medications, you are advised first to consult your health practitioner before making any changes to your lifestyle and diet.

British Library Cataloguing in Publication Data: a CIP record of this book is available from the British Library.

Print ISBN: 978-1-78161-130-2
Ebook ISBN: 978-1-78161-131-9

Editor: Georgina Bentliff
Cover design: Sylvia Kwan
Illustrations and cover image: Rolo Ledesma
Text designed and typeset: Julie Bennett
Index: Dr Laurence Errington
Production: Helen Whitehorn of Path Projects Ltd
Printed and bound: TJ International Ltd, Cornwall, UK

Contents

About the authors

The author

Bernard Raxlen BA, MD, PhD
Dr Raxlen obtained a BA in philosophy and anthropology from Stanford University. It was there he was influenced by his professor, Gregory Bateson, the noted anthropologist who introduced him to 'general systems theory' (see Chapter 11), medical ethnology and communication theory. As a result, during his medical training at the University of Toronto, Dr Raxlen worked two full summers in Quetzaltenango, Guatemala, and San Salvador, assisting medical personnel in helping native Indian people in both countries. He completed an internship at McGill Medical School Hospital Network. He then worked a full year in the emergency room of a large Toronto hospital, as well as serving as an associate 'medical house call doctor'.

His interest in medical anthropology in underdeveloped countries took him to Belem, Brazil, and the Amazon River, where he spent a year in the Xingu River Basin. He lived with an indigenous Amazonian tribe for six months. There he studied parasitology and other tropical diseases. This resulted in a life-long interest in therapeutic herbal medicine.

He returned the following year to begin training at the University of Chicago Medical School. He received a two-year advanced fellowship in Family and Child Psychiatry. He was appointed to the faculty as a lecturer in Family and Child Psychiatry.

His practice moved to Connecticut in 1972 where he was appointed lecturer at Fairfield University and Assistant Clinical

Professor in the Department of Psychiatry at Yale University. In 1975, he was appointed Director of the Children's Service Center of Bridgeport and founded the Graduate Center for Clinical Studies at the University of Bridgeport.

After a decade of private practice (1978-1988) pioneering nutritional and integrative psychiatry/medicine, he became interested in tick-borne disease (Lyme disease) because of the chronic undiagnosed symptoms of his patients.

Dr Raxlen's practice was situated in the highly Lyme endemic areas of Westchester and Fairfield counties. Over the past 15 years, he has successfully treated over 3500 cases of tick-borne disease, specializing in neuropsychiatric and neurocognitive complications. Over 90 per cent of his practice is now devoted entirely to chronic Lyme disease (CLD) and co-infections.

The diagnosis and treatment of tick-borne disease (TBD) are complicated and require not only clinical observation but also modern medical technology. This includes utilization of advanced radiology (SPECT and MRI), comprehensive neuropsychiatric evaluation (testing), serology from specialty laboratories, advanced co-infection testing (for Babesia, Bartonella and Ehrlichia/Anaplasma), sleep lab assessment and physical therapy evaluation. Presently, Dr Raxlen is one of the few family psychiatrists in the tri-state area to initiate a total comprehensive treatment program which utilizes both oral and intravenous (IV) antibiotic treatment. He also uses other treatment strategies such as neuropharmacology and stress management for:

- depression
- panic disorder
- bipolar mood disorder
- epileptiform seizure activity
- ADD
- memory loss
- sleep disorder and pre-frontal lobe deficit syndrome.

He employs nutriceutical supplements to support the patient's natural immunologic healing system.

He was an original member and co-founder of AIMS (Academy for Integrated Medical Studies) and served for several years on the Board of Directors of the Omega Institute. He was a founding member of ILADS, and was elected secretary of the first board of governors of ILADS (the International Lyme and Associated Disease Society). He has been a featured speaker in more than 40 workshops over the years on topics ranging from psychiatry, drug abuse, psychoneuroimmunology and tick-borne diseases. He has been on national television (ABC, NBC, Fox) discussing the medical concerns which pertain to TBD. Dr Raxlen is featured on the Discovery Channel in the Mystery Illness discussing Lyme Disease and its diagnosis.

With:

Allie Cashel

Allie Cashel is the author of *Suffering the Silence: Chronic Lyme Disease in an Age of Denial* (North Atlantic Books) and is the co-founder and president of The Suffering the Silence Community, a non-profit organization dedicated to breaking the stigma surrounding chronic illness and disability. Since starting work with STS, Allie has been invited to facilitate workshops and to speak about disability, inclusion and storytelling at events around the country. She has appeared in a number of global media outlets, including Good Day NY (Fox5) and NowThis Live News, and has presented her work at a United States Congressional Forum.

Alongside her advocacy work in the illness and disability community, Allie works as a marketing and content development consultant for non-profit and mission-driven companies in the United States and Europe.

Harnessing the power of storytelling, she gives voice to individuals and organizations working to create positive change in the world. Allie graduated from Bard College in 2013 with a BA in Written Arts and lives in Burlington, Vermont.

Contributing authors

Laura Alonso Canal MD (Chapter 17)
Dr Laura Alonso is a Pediatrician in Madrid. She also has experience in the treatment of adults. She studied Medicine in the Complutense University of Madrid followed by two years of residency in Internal Medicine in Barcelona with an emphasis on infectious diseases. She completed the four-year specialty training in Pediatrics at the Niño Jesús Hospital and has a Masters Degree in Tropical Medicine. She is devoted to the treatment of Lyme disease in its many manifestations and has a special interest in pediatric gastroenterology, performing upper and lower endoscopies in children. She searches for underlying infections in autistic children and in children with inflammatory bowel disease. Dr Alonso uses nutritional therapy for many of her patients together with antibiotic and herbal treatments. She firmly believes in the important role that underlying infections play nowadays in neurodegenerative, psychiatric and autoimmune disorders.

Jennifer Armstrong BSc, MD, DIBEM (Chapter 21)
Dr Jennifer Armstrong founded the Ottawa Environmental Health Clinic, in the capital of Canada in 1997 to treat environmentally ill patients. She was expecting to be treating patients made ill by the environment with chronic symptoms such as fatigue, chemical sensitivities, asthma, obesity etc, and was doing well, but eventually, as the first five years passed realized that the patients she was unable to help had tick- and other vector-borne illnesses. Utilizing techniques such as detoxification, diet, nutritional supplements and environmental adjustments along with antibiotics and herbs , her patients are generally able to attain wellness. Ottawa has become a hot spot for Lyme in Canada and there are many patients who need help. She believes that it is important to be patient-centered and diversified in how to use the available science to diagnose and treat these vector-

borne illnesses and that in time the rest of the community will understand that these patients can get better and there can be help for them.

Michael Cook (Chapter 14)

Michael J Cook, born in 1943 in Redcar, England, graduated with a BSc degree from London University (Physics and Mathematics). His career was in the semiconductor/computer chip industry working in the UK, US and for a US/Japanese joint venture over a period of 36 years. Initially working in research and development of process technology he moved into engineering management, directing research and production teams in the US, Europe and Asia.

He retired to the south coast of England in 1999 where, after a few years of various severe and recurring medical problems, he was diagnosed with Lyme disease in 2009. Since then he has applied his analytical skills to investigate many aspects of the disease. This resulted in the first publication of an investigation of the commonly stated claim that it requires 24 or 48 hours of tick attachment for transmission of Lyme disease in 2015. The original source of this claim and its inaccuracy was presented. He is co-author of a meta-analysis of the accuracy of commercial test kits for Lyme disease, published in 2016, and developed an algorithm that extended Bayes theorem which was used in two co-authored papers that quantified the accuracy of the two-tier test methodology widely recommended by most medical authorities for diagnosis of Lyme disease, and demonstrated the high levels of false negative tests.

He has made presentations of his work at conferences in Paris and Boston as well as to the members of the UK House of Commons, medical, local government and environmental and health agencies. He works as an advocate for Lyme patients and carried out a technical investigation of a UK Lyme reference laboratory where a number of short-comings were detected and the facility closed. He is a trustee of the Vis a Vis Symposium charity which brings experts from around the world to speak to UK medical professionals, and continues to work on many aspects of Lyme and related tick-borne diseases.

Doug Fearn (Chapter 4)
Doug Fearn is President of the Lyme Disease Association of Southeastern Pennsylvania, Inc. He was first officially diagnosed with Lyme disease in 1994, but he was almost certainly infected long before. Living in a semi-rural area of Chester County, Pennsylvania, prompted him to begin saving articles on Lyme disease back in the 1980s. His worst long-term symptom has been unrelenting fatigue, which has often made his life as a small business owner difficult. Both his wife and daughter have also been infected.

Doug was involved with several Lyme patient groups over the years, and in 1999 he wrote the booklet, *Lyme Disease: The Basics* which is now in its seventh edition and has been requested by over 400,000 people. In 2003 he and several other Lyme patients formed the Lyme Disease Association of Southeastern Pennsylvania, Inc., which is dedicated to education, support, and prevention of tick-borne diseases.

He has given over 300 presentations on Lyme disease to community groups, schools, deer forums, legislators, medical professionals and businesses. He has provided testimony to government agencies at the township, state and federal level. He is a member of the International Lyme and Associated Diseases Society (ILADS), a professional medical organization. In 2004, he designed a study that surveyed the population of a small township in Chester County, which revealed that nearly a quarter of the population had been diagnosed and treated for Lyme disease, and a third of those people still suffered symptoms. The results were provided to the county and state health departments, and a poster presentation was published at the 2004 ILADS conference.

John Lambert MD PhD (Chapter 15)
Dr Lambert is a consultant in Medicine and Infectious Diseases (MD PhD) at the Mater Public and Private Hospitals and Rotunda Hospitals, Dublin, Ireland, and teaches at the UCD (University College Dublin) School of Medicine and Medical Science. He qualified in New York State and was involved in evaluating and diagnosing many Lyme disease patients. In addition, during his time at Johns Hopkins in Baltimore, he was involved in the evaluation of a then soon to be licensed Lyme Vaccine and was a member of the Data Safety and Monitoring Board for this vaccine. During his 24 years as an infectious diseases consultant he has been diagnosing and treating Irish patients with Lyme infections and co-infections contracted within Ireland and more commonly Irish patients who acquired these infections abroad.

Jenna Luché-Thayer, MIA (Chapter 23)
Jenna Luché-Thayer is founder and Director of the Ad Hoc Committee for Health Equity in ICD11 Borreliosis Codes. She is a former Senior Advisor to the US Government and the United Nations and is currently assisting institutions and communities in building a humane and rights-based patient-centered response to the global borreliosis pandemic. Luché-Thayer has 33 years of policy and grassroots experience in 42 countries and works across the globe to help institutions remedy entrenched practices of discrimination that interfere with their higher purpose. Her expertise includes government transparency, accountability, human rights and political representation of marginalized groups.

Luché-Thayer has worked with governments, the United Nations, non-profits and the corporate world and has over 75 publications to her name. Her awards include: the International Woman's Day Award for Exemplary Dedication and Contributions to Improving the Political and Legal Status of Women (US government), Highest Ranking Technical Area in Accomplishment, Innovation and Comparative Advantage for the United Nations Capital Development Fund, and the

International Lyme and Associated Diseases Society Power of Lyme Award 2018. (www.gnid.world)

Mualla McManus BSc(Hons), MSc, BPharm, PhD, MBA, MPSA, AACP, FPGA (Chapter 20)
Dr Mualla McManus instigated the formation of the Tick Borne Diseases Unit at the School of Medical Sciences (Pharmacology), University of Sydney. Through her insight, Australia was re-awakened to the presence of tick-borne diseases and their impact on health.

She is the founding director of the Karl McManus Foundation (www.kmf.org.au) and Karl McManus Institute, Director of Gold Cross Pharmacy and About Redfern Medical Centre in Redfern NSW. She was pivotal in the formation of the Clinical Advisory Committee on Lyme disease, advising the Chief Medical Officer of Australia. She graduated from Monash University with Honours in immunology, MSc in cancer biology from University of Melbourne, BPharm from Monash University and PhD in neurosciences from the University of Sydney. She was a postdoctoral fellow at the Garvan Institute, Sydney. She has published in peer review journals on the impact of tick-borne diseases on the immune system and the ramifications for testing. She is active in research into tick-borne diseases, advocating for patients and liaising with all stakeholders to get a better understanding of tick/arthropod-borne diseases in the world.

Zhaneta Misho (Chapter 18)
Zhaneta Misho is the founder of the Misho Natural Healing Centre. With a tried and tested combination of scientific approaches and natural healing methods, she accompanies her patients on their individual journey to health. In her 30 years as a health practitioner she has acquired a great variety of additional therapeutic qualifications. As a specialist for complementary cancer therapy, orthomolecular medicine and TCM (Acupuncture Diploma A) she helps her patients to reach lasting improvements

in their personal energy levels and quality of life. In addition, she is deeply committed to making her field more accessible to physicians and natural health practitioners by organizing events and workshops.

Omar Morales MD (Chapter 22)
Dr Omar Morales is the Founder of Lyme Disease Mexico. He developed a special interest in treating tropical diseases with a hematological approach while living in Puerto Vallarta. While dealing with a challenging case of severe Babesia and other co-infections, Dr Morales was able to utilize his transfusion medicine background and blood bank resources to implement a novel way of treating this particular patient. Red blood cell transfusions proved to be a successful way of eradicating Babesia. This led Dr Morales to continue learning and advancing intricate protocols to address Lyme disease and other co-infections. He continues to be an active researcher of the renowned Centro Biomedical de Occidente as well as contributing to many publications, both internationally and nationally. He strongly believes that with effective medical research and analysis, eventually the majority of the healthcare community will agree that to meet as big a challenge as Lyme disease, a multidisciplinary and integrative approach will be the only way.

Christian Perronne MD, PhD (Chapter 16)
Dr Christian Perronne qualified in Internal Medicine and is Professor of Infectious and Tropical Diseases at the University of Versailles-St Quentin, Paris-Saclay, France. Since 1994, he has been head of a Department of Medicine at the Raymond Poincaré University Hospital in Garches, Greater Paris University Hospitals group. He had major responsibilities within several institutions: the Pasteur Institute in Paris (vice-director of the national tuberculosis reference center), French College of Professors of Infectious and Tropical Diseases (chairman), French National Technical Advisory Group of Experts on Immunisation

(chairman), French Drug Agency (chairman of several working groups making evidence-based recommendations), Superior Council for Public Hygiene in France (chairman), French High Council for Public Health (chairman of the Communicable Diseases Commission), INSERM, National Council of Universities (chairman for infectious and tropical diseases), and the European Advisory Group of Experts on Immunisation at the World Health Organization (vice-chairman). He has been principal investigator of several major clinical trials. He is author or co-author of more than 300 scientific publications in peer-reviewed journals. Since 1994, Christian Perronne has been involved in the management of chronic Lyme and associated diseases. He is leading a coalition of patients and physicians for the recognition of chronic Lyme disease and other crypto-infections (hidden infections) in France. He is co-founder and vice-president of the French Federation against Tick-borne Diseases (FFMVT) and president of its scientific council. He is author of a book *La Vérité sur la Maladie de Lyme* (*The Truth about Lyme Disease*), published by Odile Jacob publishers, Paris.

Armin Schwarzbach MD PhD (Chapter 19)
Dr Armin Schwarzbach, Physician, Specialist in Laboratory Medicine and founder of Armin Labs, has been at the forefront of tick-borne research for more than 20 years and is an expert in diagnosing and treating infectious diseases. He is an Advisory Board member of AONM London, England, a board member of the German Borreliosis Society and a member of the International Lyme and Associated Diseases Society (ILADS) and has served as an expert on advisory committees on Lyme disease in Australia, Canada, Ireland, France, England, Sweden and Germany.

Part One

Slipping through the cracks

To the naked eye, it is invisible, a nothing. Under the microscope it seems a silvery corkscrew undulating on a dark field. The form has simple elegance, like the whorl of a nautilus shell or the sweep of a dragonfly wing. But that simplicity is an illusion. Through the more powerful electron microscope you see not a featureless wiggle, but a shape-shifter – now a spiral, now a thread, now a rod or a sphere – with two walls, a dozen whiplike appendages and internal structures. And beyond any microscope's view, revealed only indirectly, by laboratory tests, lies a marvel of complexities. The surface bristles with molecules that sense and respond to the environment, and the interior churns like a chemical factory. Inside, more than a thousand genes flicker on and often changing sequences, to allow survival in places as different as a tick's gut, a dog's knee and a human brain.

The Biography of a Germ, Arno Karlen

Introduction

What if, at this very moment, hundreds of thousands of people were unaware that they were living in the midst of an epidemic so large that it dwarfs the AIDS epidemic by sheer numbers in North America?

What if this epidemic cut across all populations: women and men, children and adults, the infirm and the fit, the very poor and the very rich?

What if many of our best doctors in cities like New York, London, Paris, Dublin, Sydney and San Francisco were unaware of this very same problem?

This epidemic is upon us. It lurks in the most seductive of locations outside our cities – sought-after vacation places frequented by urban dwellers. These are the favorite getaway spots for the often millions of people who work in our city centers, many of whom are unaware that they are at risk of infection from this insidious microbe.

I'm talking about a tick-borne disease, namely the spirochete bacterium *Borrelia burgdorferi*, or Lyme disease, as it is more commonly known. Along with a number of other co-infectious pathogens, including deadly viruses, this bacterium has become the scourge of the Northern Hemisphere and is now reaching across Europe, into Asia and even Australia.[1]

Though the infection is spreading at unprecedented rates, the disease can be hard to spot. Its tell-tale bullseye rash only appears 25-30 per cent of the time, and sometimes three to six weeks after original exposure.[2] Other early signs and symptoms may be attributable to simple 'flu (fever, sore muscles and joints, fatigue) and often can go unnoticed. Then months, or even years, later persistent, intractable symptoms may appear, including neurological, cognitive, psychiatric, arthritic and/or musculoskeletal problems, or chronic fatigue and exhaustion. According to a study in the *American Journal of Medicine*, these patients are often as impaired as those in congestive heart failure.[3]

It should not come as a surprise, therefore, that physicians practicing in cities around the world have missed the diagnosis of an infection so enigmatic. Lyme and other tick-borne diseases have become a global scourge. Yet the medical world has been shockingly slow to react. Why is this?

Size and scale – tick-borne disease myopia

Let's take a look at New York City as a primary example of those at risk for tick-borne infection. There are 8.5 million people in New York City's five boroughs. It is estimated that approximately 20-25 per cent of the population may leave the 'concrete metropolis' for the pleasures of the natural world each year. More visit nearby parklands within the city. Other people leave the city for vacation areas in New Jersey, Connecticut, Long Island, Cape Cod, the Hudson Valley, Fire Island, Maine, and many more wooded and coastal areas. All of these locations are considered to be highly endemic areas for Lyme and other tick-borne diseases.

The Center for Disease Control in the United States recently stated that the number of individuals infected with Lyme disease is likely to be 10 times higher than has already been reported.[4] Already, this suggests that tens of thousands have been infected with Lyme over the last 10 years and have not been diagnosed. If we were to add the number of undiagnosed urban cases to that statistic, how many would we report? If we consider just 1 per cent of the number of New York travelers 'at risk', that amounts to a minimum of no less than 20,000 people infected yearly.

These numbers, on first inspection, may appear disproportionately inflated and exaggerated, but simple calculations extending over the past 10 years bring the number of cases of tick-borne disease currently undiagnosed in New York City's five boroughs to an outrageously high number.

If this is a true estimate of the problem, even by half, I find myself facing two fundamental questions: Why hasn't the sheer number of cases of tick-borne diseases (TBD) overwhelmed the general medical community here in New York, and in other medical epicenters around the world? And: Why are skilled MDs, with flawless credentials, not aware that there is a microbial complex of almost pandemic proportions affecting hundreds of their patients? No one seems to be asking these questions.

Chapter 1

Why is a psychiatrist treating Lyme disease?

Physicians located in urban centers tend to be highly respected leaders in their specialties. Like most specialists, they are trained to concentrate specifically on one part of the body. In order to operate in this 'reductionist specialist system of thought', organ systems become separated. Thus, the more specialized the physician, the more difficulty he may have recognizing a puzzling group of transient, and seemingly unrelated, symptoms.

I was trained as a psychiatrist, one of a breed of specialists often known as the 'Don Quixotes of medicine'. In spite of my specialty training, I have devoted the last 30 years of my medical practice to the treatment of tick-borne disease. An obvious question presents itself here: 'What are you doing in another specialty, namely "infectious disease"?' Let me try to answer this legitimate question as best I can.

I was rigorously trained in the scientific, evidence-based practice of diagnosis and treatment. I was taught to divide patient problems into body (physical), brain (neurological), and mind (consciousness, thoughts, emotion). This prevailing thought process is known as dualism, and is the reductionist, deductive method taught in medical schools. It is also the scientific method taught and employed by most modern medical practitioners around the world.

When the body is theoretically divided into boundaries

and systems, different symptoms become assigned to specific specialties. The brain is the province of neurologists, neurosurgeons and neuroscientists. These specialists employ impressive technology to explore the architecture, inner metabolic workings and pathology of the brain, using tools such as MRIs, CAT scans, SPECT scans, PET scans, etc.

In a somewhat different world, the psychiatrist deals with the non-physical realm of the brain, the ephemeral reality of ghosts, hallucinatory daemons, manic-depressive exaggerations, paranoid delusions, ADHD, PANDAS and neurotic Oedipal obsessions. However, the specialties of psychiatry and psychology, almost by default, also investigate spheres of cognition, consciousness, sexuality, memory, learning, creativity and emotions. In short, the specialty encompasses all that makes us distinctly human.

I consider myself, first, a medical doctor and, second, by specialty, a psychiatrist. This specialty training, and my first 10 years of active practice in psychiatry, have placed me in a unique situation when dealing with tick-borne disease.

Finding my way to tick-borne disease

I spent my first 10 years in my specialty practicing and teaching 'family systems' psychiatry, an approach that studies the family as a unit, rather than singling out a single individual. During this time, I developed a special interest in environmental medicine. I started to see, and to treat, children and adults for the effects of nutritional imbalances. These included food allergies, gluten sensitivity, hypoglycemia, mold toxicity, candida yeast, undiagnosed hypothyroid states, heavy metals and life stresses, all of which had contributed to, and provoked, mental illnesses such as anxiety, depression, ADD or ADHD, and bipolar disorders.

I sometimes referred to these troubled patients as 'dropped through the cracks patients'. These were people who had been seen by multiple specialists, but had not been helped by the orthodox medical community, and were designated 'all-in-your-head' type patients. I found I could often help these patients by treating what had been defined as psychiatric problems with functional or integrated medical techniques. The medical orthodoxy had labeled many of these symptoms as 'medically unexplained physical symptoms', or MUPS.[5] These were conditions that appeared on the surface to have no direct cause, even after extensive, sophisticated work-ups (patient assessments) using state of the art medical diagnostic techniques.

I, as a specialist in psychiatric medicine, chose to explore and practice in this medical wasteland of MUPS, along with a new group of forward-thinking doctors. In those years, 'orthomolecular psychiatry' and 'holistic medicine' were names given to medical societies that sponsored this type of thinking. In just a few years, we had been able to successfully treat many patients with new techniques adapted from pioneer medical organizations. This included using nutritional supplements, hypoglycemic diets, intravenous vitamin C/glutathione infusions, food allergy avoidance and treatment with rotation and paleo diets, and more.

Unfortunately, there remained a group of patients who continued to have many residual symptoms, and whose health did not improve significantly. And it was this group of patients that ultimately brought me face to face with the bizarre world of Lyme disease. I have adventured in this controversial, insane, but intensely rewarding, world for the past 30 years

Around 1985, the full extent of the 'Borrelia plague' was just beginning to be investigated by a number of physicians across specialties. Physicians were witnessing a strange medical phenomenon: incapacitated patients with an unusual array of multi-systemic problems and multiple symptoms. I also witnessed the same puzzling phenomenon in my practice.

Chapter 1

Physician-psychiatrist thinking

For those already familiar with tick-borne disease, it's common knowledge that the illness knows no well-defined boundaries. The infection can enter into every system of the body and mimic other medical conditions. Though the 11th International Classification of Diseases from the World Health Organization expands the definition of Lyme disease, in practice definitions used by phyicians from the Infectious Diseases Society of America (IDSA) and the Centers for Disease Control and Prevention (CDC) are far too narrow to be clinically useful. These definitions do not acknowledge the scope and strength of the infection and the way it can move from system to system with ease. We need to think outside the box when it comes to this condition, and my particular specialty helps me to do just that.

As a physician-psychiatrist, when I see significant changes in the cognitive and emotional health of my patients (when they have been previously well adjusted), I assess them not just for psychiatric issues, but also for conditions that affect the nervous system and the body as a whole. It is also critical to understand the 'subjective world' of the patient – their thoughts, level of cognition, memory, and emotional life – that has gone awry, in making an accurate diagnosis.

In my practice, patients with complicated physical and psychiatric histories, particularly from areas where Lyme is endemic, have often been discovered to have an underlying tick-borne infection. Even people with devastating dementias, such as Alzheimer's disease, on autopsy have been found to harbor Borrelia DNA and biofilm sequestered under microscope. But in most cases, these mixtures of physical and psychiatric symptoms are not recognized as tick-borne disease. Physicians, through no fault of their own, fail to recognize the syndrome.

Approximately 20 years ago, Dr Robert Bransfield, a practicing psychiatrist in New Jersey and past president of ILADS, wrote a paper entitled: 'The Neuropsychiatric Assessment of Lyme

Disease'. In it he stated that:

> *we can view Lyme disease as a stealth Phoenix – it is difficult to find and even more difficult to eradicate after it has penetrated deep into body tissue. Once late stage Lyme exists it is impossible with current technology to prove the* B. Burgdorferi *has been eradicated. Constant vigilance is therefore necessary. Years of failure to recognize, diagnose, and adequately treat these patients has led to an ever expanding epidemic of chronic Lyme disease.*

He further stated that to know Lyme disease is not only to know medicine but also neurology, psychiatry, politics, economics and law. 'The complexity of the disease challenges our scientific as well as our ethical capabilities.'

He was absolutely correct. Treating Lyme and tick-borne disease patients, I often find that I am the final stop for many of my patients. My patients are bewildered and at a loss to know how to bridge the gap between their subjective feeling that something is wrong, and what they have been told is scientific evidence that says there is not. How to help them through this space? My role as a physician is to attempt to bridge this swift river of epistemological perplexity. I attempt to link the patient to both worlds of medical thinking and to alert them to the cognitive errors which plague medicine today, and perpetuate the mind-body split. I try to show them a way to bridge both opposing banks without being stranded by discouragement, oft-times medical neglect.

The hidden epidemic

So how many patients are actually suffering from tick-borne disease? Has this disease reached epidemic proportions, not only in New England, but also throughout the northern hemisphere? Have these infections reached Europe, Australia or South Africa?

A small tick, no bigger than a tiny dot, can remain hidden on a body part, like the back of the leg, behind the ear, or even in the hairline, never to be discovered. Where this is the case, the patients would have no reason to suspect a tick-borne disease infection if they never saw a tick. So what happens to those patients? Where do they go? What happens to the people who become lost in the system, adding more and more symptoms to their list of complaints without receiving an answer? How do these patients navigate a medical landscape where many doctors are not even aware of Lyme as a possibility? What happens to the children who are infected, but never find a proper diagnosis? What happens to young women who are pregnant, and suddenly experience symptoms that no one can find the cause of? What happens to the people who have been misdiagnosed with chronic fatigue syndrome or fibromyalgia and struggle ever to get better? And, perhaps most importantly, how, and why, are so many doctors missing diagnoses that could help people go back to living normal, healthy lives?

In this book, we will seek to answer many of those questions by presenting the perspectives of patients and physicians from around the world, and exploring the reasons for the medical myopia that so often blocks the accurate diagnosis and treatment of tick-borne disease (TBD). I will share the experience of my 30 years in the field and more than 40,000 clinical hours listening to, and treating, TBD patients. And, in an effort to illuminate the scope of this problem, I will present writing and thought-leadership from other physicians and advocates around the world willing to share experiences and expertise. I have also invited a former, but now recovered, patient, the author of *Suffering the Silence: Chronic Lyme Disease in an Age of Denial*, co-collaborator and Lyme advocate, Allie Cashel to illuminate life after tick-borne disease and the difficulties encountered in the post-Lyme world. It is my hope that this book will offer unique insight into the often-confounding labyrinth of tick-borne disease, which patients often lose themselves in before ever confronting this insidious disease.

Chapter 2

The tick-borne disease commonalities

In the uncharted world of the diagnosis and treatment of tick-borne disease, particularly when it has gone undetected for years (along with other co-infections), both physicians and patients consistently struggle to find the correct course of action as they seek both an accurate diagnosis and an accurate course of treatment.

I feel it important to note that when I speak about Lyme and tick-borne disease in general, I'm not talking about the commonly known syndrome of acute Lyme disease. This is a well-documented clinical picture of an embedded tick bite, a rash (*erythema migrans*), 'flu-like fatigue, arthritis, and, in some cases, neurological symptoms, such as brain fog and Bell's palsy. These symptoms alert most physicians in Lyme-endemic areas, and even outside of those areas. Without controversy or concern, doctors are able to treat conservatively, mostly with doxycycline (100 mg) for three to six weeks.

Many tick-borne infections do not fall into the category of acute Lyme. The kaleidoscopic tick-borne disease syndrome (Lyme and co-infections) doesn't often compute with a cautious, conservative, evidence-based medical physician who prides him/herself on scientific objectivity and evidence-based medical practice. When borreliosis is combined with more than one co-infection, it often blurs the boundaries of what is recognized as the formal, CDC, clinical description of 'Lyme disease'. Added symptoms, which are applicable to other tick-borne infections, particularly those of babesiosis and bartonellosis, complicate the clinical picture for the doctor. and make a correct diagnosis difficult.

Finding the common thread

When a physician encounters a patient for the first time, a diagnostic procedure to assess the presenting problem is set in motion. Symptoms are reviewed, physical examinations performed, diagnostic laboratory blood samples drawn and, if necessary, other procedural tests performed, such as radiology (MRI, CAT scans, ultrasound, etc.). From this information, a differential diagnosis is obtained and treatment is initiated. As scientifically and technically complete as the above 'work-up' may seem, this is where many falter when dealing with tick-borne disease (TBD). Why?

Unfortunately, using the aforementioned standard procedures does not always reveal the presence of a TBD infection. We will explore the details of diagnosis in a later chapter (page 61), but, in summary, the laboratory results for Lyme disease can be unreliable and misleading. In 30-40 per cent of cases, the procedures are positive and can help to identify the infection. But in the other 60-70 per cent of cases, especially in long-standing untreated patients, the laboratory diagnosis may be missed.[6] The reason is that the standard 'Western Blot antibody assay' is unreliable and can produce false negative results – even blood samples from the same patient that are sent to different labs for validation, can show strikingly different results.[7]

This has been an issue for more than 25 years. In a 1991 study published in the *Journal of Clinical Microbiology,* researchers reported that 55 per cent of laboratories participating in the study could not accurately identify serum samples for Lyme disease patients containing antibody against *Borrelia burgdorferi*. Six years later, they revisited the study in the hopes that they would see improvement but, unfortunately, they did not. The sensitivity of testing fluctuated between 93 per cent and 75 per cent depending on the conjugate used by the participating laboratories. Decades later, we are still seeing similar inconsistencies in the blood samples sent out for Lyme testing today.[8]

Unlike many traditional specialties in medicine, in the case of this particular infection, 'negative results' do not necessarily eliminate the possibility that the patient may be infected with a tick-borne disease. And as Mary Beth Pfeiffer states in her new book, *Lyme: The First Epidemic of Climate Change*, 'If we can't even tell if they're actively infected, how can we say that they're not?'[9]

I have found that there is a set of 'common themes' that form a consistent pattern. Almost all tick-borne disease patients, independent of their age, exhibit all or most of these common themes that define these disease states. These otherwise overlooked themes can help alert practitioners as to the likelihood of tick-borne disease.

Physician awareness of these common themes is critical to successful diagnosis and treatment. Part of the reason so many physicians miss tick-borne disease diagnosis is because they're often looking in the wrong place, or not considering information which points them in the right direction. What can appear to be illuminated areas, like blood testing (ELISA and Western Blot) often return negative results, as I have said. This inhibits any further investigation, and the diagnosis is missed.

Wrong place, wrong tools

The following popular anecdote is cited to help draw attention to the dilemma of looking in the wrong place with the wrong tools.

> *The scene is a dark night, a bright street lamp, and two men. One man is walking under the streetlight in circles, head down, apparently looking for something on the ground. The second man is walking by and notices the first man as he continues to walk around*

the illuminated area. Seeing that he appears to be frustrated, the second man approaches the street lamp and calls out, 'Hey friend, you look worried. Lost something important? What's going on?'

'I lost my girlfriend's engagement ring,' the first man grumbles. 'I was going to propose tonight.'

'That's horrible!' says the second man. 'Let me help you look.' With that said, the second man follows behind the first man and begins to search the illuminated area under the street lamp. After 10 or so minutes, the second man stops, scratches his head, looks puzzled, and then asks the first man, 'Are you sure you lost the ring right around here?'

'Oh, I'm quite sure I didn't lose it around here,' replies the first man. 'I lost it in the back alley next to the bar.' At this point the second man is completely confused.

'Then why in the world are we looking over here and walking around in circles?'

'Oh, that's easy,' says the first man, leaning against the lamp post. 'It's pitch black in the alleyway where I dropped the ring. You can't see a thing. That's why I'm looking right here. The light is so much better under the lamp post!'

With the usual investigation of tick-borne disease, the patient is often left circling a lamp post without a legitimate diagnosis and correct treatment.

So, what if we revisit the anecdote and suggest an alternative ending?

The two men are standing under the street lamp. The second man has a puzzled look on his face. He shakes his head and puts his hand on the first man's shoulder.

'We can't continue walking around here in circles because the light is better. Listen,' he says, 'I have an idea. Let's go back to where you think you first lost the ring and start looking there.

Perhaps we'll have better luck.'

'I think it's a waste of time,' says the first man. 'You can't see a thing; it's pitch black.'

'Well I think I can change that. You see I have this little flashlight with an LED bulb. It's a new technology but it works like a charm in most cases.'

'Seems too small to be of much use. I don't think we'll get anywhere doing it that way. Look how bright it is here. You can see all around you,' the first man persists.

'Let's go and give it a try,' says the second man firmly.

With that, they arrive at the dark alley. The second man takes out his LED penlight and with it illuminates a large area in the unlit alleyway. Within five minutes, the first man suddenly bends down, drops to his knees and lets out a whoop.

'I found it!' he shouts. 'I found the ring! I have it!'

'Great,' smiles the second man. 'I knew we'd find it. It's all a matter of where you look, what you look at, and what kind of light you use.'

The commonalities

In my practice, I listen to the patient's initial symptoms without interruption and then take a timeline of the history of their condition. I listen for situations that I know to be 'red flags' or specific criteria for suspecting TBD disease. These red flags are recurring history patterns that have repeated themselves again and again, hundreds of times in the course of my taking a detailed two-hour history on the first visit. In addition, prior to their visit, the patient fills out a detailed and complete symptom check-list that is reviewed and discussed. These are the familiar themes or 'repeated commonalities' that have appeared regularly in most TBD cases I have treated. These repeated commonalities are very often overlooked or not considered in the diagnostic process but can be helpful clues in guiding a physician toward a correct diagnosis.

1. Endemic areas – Where have you lived? Where have you visited?

Although it may seem perfectly obvious, an important consideration is whether or not the patient has lived in, or visited, an endemic area locally or further afield. This knowledge is probably the most important single piece of information that a physician must know before he can proceed with his analysis of a potential tick-borne disease problem. Where a patient has lived previously, or where a patient has visited, should be one of the cornerstones of the medical diagnosis of tick-borne disease.[10]

In the anecdote above, the ring was found by shifting the restricted paradigm to 'thinking outside the box'. In other words, incorporating new facts and taking a broader look at the problem. To find the ring they needed to look in the right place with the right light. When physicians do not explore the ecological environment and travel history of the patient, important diagnostic information is missed.

2. Animals – Do you, or have you had, animals that go inside or outside your living quarters?

Because of their consistent contact with their owners in domestic spaces, pets are highly suspicious tick-carriers. Dogs and cats that spend time outdoors and indoors, lying on sofas, beds and rugs, should be considered highly suspect. If they have had tick-borne disease, diagnosed by the veterinarian, then the chances greatly increase that the human patient has had exposure to an infected tick.

3. Vacations and hotspots – Have you visited vacation sites in high endemic areas at home or abroad?

Cities surrounded by a plethora of natural resources may represent a double-edged sword. The fact is that those natural resources are both favorite vacation spots and, at the same time, potential areas of infected tick ecology. The strong possibility of vacationers being infected is not really a question of 'if' but of 'when'.[11]

Even smaller day trips to favorite locations are potential visits to 'tick-borne disease territory'. Physicians need be aware of these high endemic areas surrounding their cities when taking a history from an atypical patient who just doesn't seem to fit neatly into any one diagnostic category.

Individuals also need to be cognizant of the dangers that lurk in these highly trafficked vacation hot spots. These tick-infested areas increase the chance of tick-borne disease exposure for all people visiting these places.

Although certain areas around the United States, Europe and the rest of the world are more endemic for tick-borne infection than others, it is important to know that the prevalence of ticks and Lyme disease is spreading. Ticks in certain areas, such as the American Northeast and Midwest, seem to spread the Lyme bacteria more easily than ticks in other areas. This suggests that subtle genetic differences in the ticks themselves will likely have an effect on the spread of Lyme disease and other tick-borne infections around the world.[12]

4. Have you lived in or visited property that has known deer grazers?

In many locations in the northern hemisphere, deer have become ubiquitous. Because of the pressure of advancing suburbia, the deer are increasingly forced into ecological niches, areas of suburban landscape which now host hordes of deer. Passing through walkways between houses and roaming in back yards/gardens, deer herds now regularly occupy human areas in many parts of North America. As the deer graze in human habitats and occupy smaller and smaller ecological systems, they also become ubiquitous infected-tick carriers on family properties. And since there are no natural predators to cull the deer population, this problem has exploded exponentially and unnaturally. These attractive animals bring with them, unfortunately, unrestrained destruction of personal property, serious road traffic accidents, and ever more likelihood of exposure to infected ticks.

Birds also present a unique carrier pattern in the tick ecology as suburbia advances.[13] They are present throughout the life cycle of the tick, often having direct contact with adult ticks along with the larva, nymph, and egg bunch stages (see page 36 for the Life cycle of ticks). They nest in tall grasses and feed in locations that are endemic for ticks and Lyme infection. It's also important to note that ticks at any stage of their growth (including eggs) can attach to birds' bodies.

Though many birds, like deer, are territorial and remain in one location, others are migrants. Migrating birds can fly thousands of miles to seasonal territories, spreading and mixing infected tick populations, and bringing with them increased incidence of tick-borne disease.[14]

5. Multiple visits to the doctor

One of the most common themes in a tick-borne disease patient's history is his/her visits to multiple specialists. Their history begins with a set of symptoms that wax and wane and can move from system to system. Often times, the patient will seek out their primary care doctor, who may or may not be able to recognize the possibility of tick-borne disease. Blood testing may be done, often with negative results. The patient may or may not have treatment for acute TBD (usually three to four weeks of the antibiotic doxycycline). Symptoms may persist and the patient may or may not improve.

If symptoms do not improve, or as symptoms change, the patient is referred to another specialist. And then another. Each specialist in turn does a complex work-up. These specialists include rheumatologists, internal medicine physicians, infections disease specialists, ENT specialists, physiologists and endocrinologists. It is not unusual for the patients to have seen on average nine or 10 specialists in an attempt to find a plausible diagnosis for their condition.

It's important to understand that many of these undiagnosed patients have suffered not only the debilitating physical symptoms of tick-borne disease, but also the indignity of being humiliated and demeaned by many of the specialists they have visited. These doctors will simply have doubted their veracity, or have offered diagnoses of fibromyalgia, chronic fatigue syndrome, MUPS (medically unexplained physical symptoms), chronic anxiety or depression.

A negative process, sustained by a punishing medical system, has traumatized these patients. Their self-esteem and confidence in the legitimacy of their illness will have all but been destroyed by their negative medical encounters. At best, they will have been misdiagnosed and treated for symptoms only. They will have walked away with prescriptions for multiple medications from multiple specialists in a failed attempt to reduce their symptoms. Sometimes patients will be taking six or seven different drugs at the same time when they first visit my office.

Many patients have commented that because of such a toxic response to their illness, this negative interaction has provoked a PTSD-like syndrome. These individuals will have become fearful of believing or trusting most doctors and disdain the medical profession. As a result, they just stop seeking medical help, turn to other resources, or just give up trying to find answers and live with their symptoms.

6. Objective vs. subjective symptoms

One of the hallmarks of chronic tick-borne disease patients is that they very often appear healthy but have multiple complaints. Physical examinations can be completely negative, as can their blood analyses, including Western Blot testing.[15] In spite of these apparently normal findings, they have major complaints, even debilitating symptoms, such as fatigue, exhaustion and serious joint and memory problems. Their fatigue symptoms are so intense, at times, that even a single expenditure of energy (walking the dog/cooking a meal) sends them to bed. It often takes several days to recover before they can normalize another day.

In spite of the extreme fatigue, patients also suffer from severe 'insomnia', having difficulties in both falling asleep and/or staying asleep. Sleep studies may show generalized restlessness, but not much more.[16] Yet the insomnia can be profound, and if accompanied by drenching night sweats and air hunger, there is a strong likelihood that the patient is suffering from an infection by a red-blood-cell parasite – babesiosis (see page 45) along with borreliosis.

7. Neurocognitive decline

Serious reductions in mental functioning are constants that help identify TBD patients. Almost universally, they complain of brain fog, memory loss, stuttering, confused episodes, getting lost, and seriously diminished speed of processing. Neuropsychological testing reveals often-serious dysfunction in mental processing.[17]

Individual patients, often accompanied by a spouse or family member, admit to the fact that their personalities have undergone drastic changes. Often describing themselves as ordinarily upbeat, optimistic, outgoing, socially engaged and level headed, they admit to a 'personality shift'. They don't recognize themselves. They complain that they are not presently who they were in the past. Now they are irritable, disagreeable, withdrawn, antisocial and up-tight. They openly admit to being a different person from who they were before their illness. They have visited psychiatrists, undergone therapy; have taken prescribed antidepressants and anti-anxiety agents with minimal success. They have been unable to return to their upbeat personality in spite of their best efforts.

Along with these personality changes there are also significant 'life changes', the common ones including having to drop out of college, taking disability leave from work, moving back with parents, and giving up apartments.

8. Previous TBD diagnosis/post-treatment TBD syndrome diagnosis

It is not uncommon for a patient to have had a previous diagnosis of Lyme disease (usually early acute) and treatment with doxycycline doses of 100 mg for two to four weeks. The patient may have had a varying response to that treatment, ranging from the clearing of symptoms to no change in the condition at all. A second course of antibiotics will often have continued this pattern. Sometimes, patients will have experienced neurological symptoms and have had a blood test.[18] Intravenous (IV) antibiotics will have been prescribed, usually for one month. Treatment guidelines from the Infectious Diseases Society of America (IDSA) take exception to the concept of chronic Lyme and recommend only one month of IV therapy. Should the patient have continued with their symptoms, they will have been redefined as having a 'post-Lyme syndrome' and the acute infection considered as treated.

Patients who fall into this category often are concerned about the risks of antibiotic use. They don't believe that they are well, but they worry about over-use of, and resistance to, antibiotics. Many have read editorials and popular commentaries that 'chronic Lyme' does not exist. Yet they feel something is drastically wrong with their health. They are sure that their treatments have been incomplete since many of their initial symptoms still persist at the time of their initial visit to my clinic.

Unfortunately, it has been demonstrated consistently that short-term therapies in chronic persistent tick-borne disease are not effective. Numerous studies have shown that the organisms carried by the ticks can persist after treatment. Identical symptoms that remain after the supposed treatment has been effectively concluded are then reclassified as 'post-treatment

Lyme syndrome', as I have said. Reclassifying persistent symptoms as an entirely new entity appears to be an illogical sleight-of-hand, reshuffled construct.[19]

9. Extensive experience with naturopathic medicine/doctors

Patients who have been dismissed by their physicians without a diagnosis may turn to non-physician practitioners. In particular, they will turn to chiropractors, naturopaths, homeopaths, herbalists, nutritionists and other auxiliary practitioners for advice. Some patients have been definitely helped by these consultations.

One reason simply is that the sufferers have been listened to empathically by these professionals. Natural remedies, diet change and detoxification protocols have also helped many patients. However, these patients often bring bags full of supplements to their initial visit (vitamins, herbs, natural sleep medicines, anti-inflammatory products etc). They appear confused as to whether these products have helped their symptoms and the course of their disease. They don't know if they are making them better or making them worse. They may have tried acupuncture, colonics, detox footbaths, Raki healing, ozone, IV vitamin infusions, Reif machines – all in an effort to improve symptoms. While these treatments will often help support patient healing, they rarely get to the root of the problem if this is a persistent infection.

10. Internet surfing

Out of frustration at not being helped or understood by the orthodox medical community, many patients will take it upon themselves to search for answers to their condition themselves. They often come into my office armed with information gleaned from the internet. They will have accessed the Facebook pages of other suffering patients, have discussed their problem with fellow Lyme journeymen, have read numerous Lyme books, and have responded to numerous websites promising herbal and other 'natural' cures. They will have acquired information about their possible Lyme diagnosis and will be sure they have the disorder. Often times they will have strong ideas as to how they should be treated and what combinations of medications should be used.

They will also bring with them indeterminate laboratory results, including Lyme testing, which increases their suspicions of a possible connection between their longstanding symptoms and a diagnosis of tick-borne disease.

This picture should be considered a 'red flag'. It is usually a sign that these patients have been struggling on their own to try and understand their complex illness. Very often they are impatient to know that their interpretation of their condition is correct. They will be insistent on getting answers to the seriousness of their chronic symptoms and impatient to initiate treatment as quickly as possible.

This type of patient will irritate most specialists and, with a negative work-up and sero-negative laboratory results, they will be quickly dismissed as NLD ('not Lyme disease') and left again to their own resources. The repetitive behavior will begin anew. Desperate for a Lyme diagnosis to explain their chronic illness, the patient will return again to his/her only source of information, security and hope of a cure – namely, the highly inconsistent and often unreliable internet.

11. Family dynamics and simultaneous infections

In the early part of my career in psychiatry I was trained in family systems therapy, as I have said. Family systems therapy is the approach that the therapist sees the whole family as a unit, rather than singling out a designated individual. I have integrated that experience with my work in the tick-borne disease field and have seen a countless number of family members over my 30 years in practice. I have been struck by the terrible toll tick-borne diseases extact on the wellbeing and dynamics of the family as a whole.

Multiple members of the same family may be infected – mothers and fathers, sisters and brothers – often unaware, all at the same time. Or they may be infected at different times over the course of many years. All the members of the same family may have suffered from exposure to Lyme and other tick-borne disease at one time or another, some with extreme symptoms, others almost asymptomatic.

These multiple bacteriological strains that debilitate the individual can create chaos in the family system. Each individual may be struggling differently with the effects of their infection at the same time. Empathy, understanding and patience can wear thin within the family as the disease becomes chronic. Months, even years, pass with the symptoms becoming intractable. The result may be emotional distancing of family members. Unfortunately, when there is no definitive diagnosis or treatment forthcoming from multiple specialists, members of the family become alienated and may split apart, ending in separation, or even worse, divorce.

I will add that when children who have been emotionally well-balanced and happy suddenly appear to have been affected by a mood disorder (such as atypical bipolar disorder of childhood) or a non-specific psychiatric illness, oppositional disorder, or even ADHD, the physician or family must be alerted to the possibility of infection, inflammation and neurological disruption brought on by a tick-borne disease.

12. Red flag symptoms

The following specific 'red flag' symptoms regularly appear in patients infected with tick-borne disease:

- Embedded tick
- Bullseye rash (Borrellia)
- Shortness of breath (Babesia)

- Air hunger and negative pulmonary function examination (Babesia)
- Drenching night sweats (Babesia)
- Swollen joints (Borrelia)
- Light sensitivity (Borrelia and Bartonella)
- Sound sensitivity (Borrelia and Bartonella)
- Touch sensitivity (Borrelia and Bartonella)
- Plantar fasciitis (painful heel / sole of foot) (Bartonella)
- Sudden psychiatric or neurocognitive impairment (Borellia and Bartonella)
- Unprovoked nausea (Bartonella)
- Sudden panic attacks and unprovoked anxiety (Borrelia and Bartonella)
- Purple / red streaks or scratches (Bartonella)
- New episodes of migraine headaches (Borrelia)
- Decreased hearing in one or both ears; idiopathic hearing loss (Borrelia)
- Sudden and persistent insomnia (Borrelia)
- Gastrointestinal symptoms (Bartonella)
- Vagus nerve neuropathies (Borrelia)
- Cardiovascular abnormalities: POTS (postural orthostatic tachycardia syndrome), tachycardia, bundle branch block, palpitations and missed heart beats (Borrelia)
- Strange, persistent symptoms:
    - gravity pulling patient into the floor
    - constant sweating on one side of the body
    - numbness from the waist down
    - confusion of day-to-day acts
    - inability to recognize friends' and family's faces
    - psychogenic or emotionally driven seizures
    - symptom free and then sudden onset of multi-system complaints
    - de-personalization (a sense of being outside one's body / being separated from the world by a glass barrier)

- loss of reading ability
- loss of mathematic abilities
- depth perception issues
- gradual changes in vision without an ophthalmological diagnosis
- sudden irrational suicidal thoughts (turning one's car into oncoming traffic, jumping from a bridge)
- sudden irrational homicidal thoughts (killing one's children)

- Migrating pain, particularly in joints, muscles, and nerves that may be here one day, gone tomorrow.

The above *repeated commonalities* should be vital clues for the clinician in the diagnosis of TBD. The results of laboratory Western Blot or other serum tests must be carefully weighed against the 'suspicious index' of the above categories. To disregard the likelihood of a tick-borne infection solely on the basis of an indeterminate or negative Western Blot by CDC standards, in my view, is tantamount to malpractice. This list of clinical clues should accompany the patient on his/her consultation with his/her family physician or specialist in order to discuss intelligently the possibility of TBD.

The reality of our current situation, however, is that many of these repeated commonalities are not used to diagnose TBD, but are instead over-looked or even sometimes used to make the NLD ('not Lyme disease') diagnosis. As briefly mentioned above, I believe it is the failure of our traditional diagnosis process that makes this possible.

Searching for repeated commonalities and completing a comprehensive patient history will always be vital pieces of the TBD diagnosis puzzle, but if we could repair that first step – find a solution for the failed testing – it would be significantly easier for the mainstream medical community accurately to diagnose, and even accept, the climbing numbers of infected patients.

Chapter 3

Recognition of tick-borne disease

Due to the fact that physicians so often miss the diagnosis of tick-borne disease (TBD) as the root cause of patient suffering, many individuals who should be considered 'at risk' for infection are instead labeled with another 'non-specific' diagnosis. In a sense, they are left in a holding pattern, with 'symptoms' and not 'causes' being treated indefinitely. Eager to help, specialists will refer the patient from colleague to colleague, often with minimal results.

In these cases, often in frustration, the unsuspecting physician wishing to put diagnostic closure on those diverse symptoms will attach various descriptive labels to fit the unwell patient: fibromyalgia, chronic fatigue syndrome, chronic viral syndrome, depression, stress or 'seasonal affective disorder with migraine headaches', are some of the more common 'diagnoses'.

Surprisingly, these diagnoses are often easier to make than a Lyme diagnosis – even with a positive blood result. Why? These 'syndromes' include a much larger, encompassing list of symptoms that can be used to make a diagnosis. One could argue that the biggest impediment to the recognition of tick-borne disease, and as a result the tick-borne disease epidemic, are the strict 'symptom criteria' for reporting a new case. The skepticism surrounding Lyme and 'chronic Lyme' in the mainstream medical world also makes a diagnosis challenging. Patients living with long-term tick-borne infections are often dismissed as having a diagnosis entitled 'post-treatment Lyme syndrome' or PTLS. This is a syndrome that suggests that patients who have received any treatment for Lyme or TBD do not have active infection, but instead are exhibiting 'medically unexplained' symptoms (MUPS).

Skeptics of Lyme and chronic infection often point to certain diagnosis trends to prove that 'chronic Lyme disease' is not a 'real thing'. For example, some have recently pointed to gender imbalance in CDC diagnoses, which are disproportionately female. In an article entitled 'The Science Isn't Settled on Chronic Lyme', Maya Dusenbery and Julie Rehmyer explain this thinking, stating that gender imbalance in diagnosis statistics brought skeptics to the conclusion that 'Lyme must be "unrelated to infection with *B. burgdorferi*",' and instead consists of misdiagnosis of 'illnesses with a female preponderance, such as fibromyalgia, chronic fatigue syndrome, or depression'.[20]

In the United States, the Centers for Disease Control and Prevention (CDC) is the leading national public health institute and the organization responsible for reporting the number of infectious disease cases in the country each year. The symptom criteria for reporting Lyme disease were accepted by the CDC in the mid-1970s, when the condition was first being reported in the American Northeast.[21] At the time, these criteria were intended for statistical purposes only, and not for making a clinical diagnosis. In other words, as they were originally intended, the CDC diagnostic guidelines for tick-borne disease should never be used by doctors or patients, only by epidemiologists and statisticians.

Though the World Health Organization (WHO) and the the International Lyme and Associated Diseases Society (ILADS) have both moved on to update their treatment guidelines, unfortunately for the CDC, 'time has stood still' on their version of the guidelines. Doctors around the world still use these every day in the diagnosis process, but the organization has never updated their reporting 'Lyme case' guidelines. They most certainly have never gone any further in elucidating what symptoms constitute an 'active clinically positive Lyme patient'. There is still a highly skewed and absurdly 'exclusive limited definition' on how this disease is expressed symptomatically and clinically, making it nearly impossible for our overworked and time-pressed physicians to 'get it right'.

In spite of more than 40 years of research and evolving theory in the field of tick-borne disease, acceptance has been incredibly slow for the governmental institutions that inform diagnosis and treatment by physicians. Their intransigence is similar to insisting on driving a 'horse-and-buggy' for daily transportation in today's highly trafficked NYC. Modern cars whizz past from all directions, yet the CDC and Infectious Diseases Society of America (IDSA) still insist on blatantly ignoring progress and blithely bump along in their antiquated buggies. They carefully select or exclude contradictory science, or specifically limit significant input from outside sources, such as patient groups, physicians who are actively engaged in treating TBD, new updated treatment guidelines from the International Lyme and Associated Diseases Society (ILADS) and published scientific research.

Fortunately, this is beginning to change. Over the past 10 years, leaders from ILADS have repeatedly reached out to medical journals and to governments to express concern over the practices and guidelines laid out by the CDC and IDSA. In one letter to the *American Journal of Medicine* referring to opinion pieces citing the CDC and IDSA guidelines, my colleagues Raphael Stricker and Lorraine Johnson wrote: 'Among the more than 25,000 peer-reviewed articles on tick borne disease listed on the PubMed database, there are literally hundreds that contradict the selective "evidence" that these opinion pieces are willing to acknowledge… The political problem with this series of opinion pieces is that they gloss over the shortcomings of the shaky IDSA Lyme guidelines that have recently come under attack in scientific and legislative investigations.'[22]

Physicians themselves are well aware of these shortcomings. My colleague, Dr Robert Bransfield, conducted a physician's opinion survey of licensed physicians who evaluate and treat patients with tick-borne disease to compare the credibility of the IDSA guidelines with the ILADS guidelines. Fifty respondents from 19 different states and two different countries who have experience in treating a total of 374,683 cases of Lyme disease were surveyed. There was a 100 per cent consensus that there is a controversy over the standard of care for this condition.

Altogether 98 per cent of the physicians surveyed stated that the ILADS guidelines better address the full range of Lyme and TBD presentation and better reflect future directions for treatment; 88 per cent of participants also stated that the ILADS guidelines better represent an impartial view of the literature on TBD, and 90 per cent reported that they appeared less biased than the IDSA guidelines.[23]

The Federal government has convened a task force, divided into a number of different sub-groups, to investigate all aspects of this worldwide pandemic. This includes contributions from IDSA and ILADS treating physicians, research scientists, patient activists, laboratory pathologists and heads of infectious disease departments from prestigious universities. WHO has also released the 11th International Classification of Diseases which provides a much broader and more in-depth look at the complexities of Lyme and TBD.

These organizations have explored such important issues as inadequate or inconsistent testing, sero-negative active Lyme (that is, where there are symptoms but the blood test is negative), new testing concepts, co-infections, cognitive issues and changes, childhood TBD, neurologic issues (psychiatric syndromes, multiple sclerosis, ALS, Parkinsons, congenital Lyme and autism), and persistent or chronic Lyme disease treated with extended antibiotic protocols. Despite this, they have all been systematically ignored by the CDC and IDSA.

This lack of systematic acceptance for the scale and scope of the Lyme epidemic also contributes to the tens of thousands of individuals who are left without a diagnosis, or in many cases, with a diagnosis that does not reflect their experience of illness and disease. As stated by Dusenbery and Rehmeyer, 'the skeptics act as though the science is already settled, when in actuality, patients are suffering desperately for lack of science.'[24]

Along with physicians from countries in Europe, Canada, Mexico, USA and Australia, I have over the years taken a special interest in those lost or 'fallen-through-the-cracks' patients, who experience a life-changing illness but face a diagnostic blind alley. We physicians have come to understand that the treatment of TBD, for all practical purposes, has become a 'new medical subspecialty since its symptomatology is so ubiquitous and extends into all systems. I think we look upon this emerging field as a special challenge. We have the opportunity to provide care for a large and diverse group of neglected patients, in need of serious medical attention. Unfortunately, in too many instances, the larger medical community has taken a skeptical and dismissive approach to these people. However, with the application of correct treatment, many emotionally and physically exhausted individuals in my practice undergo a positive and dramatic change in their health. Their debilitating symptoms over time are significantly reduced, their condition is considerably improved, and they are able to return to their previously normal routines, at work, at home and at play.

The stories of these people and their journeys through the TBD labyrinth are important ones in that these patients represent a new subspecialty. In them we can find details about the complex landscape of the tick-borne disease epidemic.

In writing this book, I have chosen to use a creative method that I refer to as a 'medical intuitive narrative' (MIN). I have tried to highlight typical cases of TBD that I encounter daily in my practice. Instead of quoting directly from a patient's case record, which you can find examples of in the appendix, I have attempted to create a different format to bring to life the actual 'lived reality' of each patient.

Chapter 3

Every story that you will read in the next section represents the type of patient and the type of case that passes through my office, and the offices of many the other physicians in this book who treat these conditions, every day.

In order to make these cases represent 'real life', rather than a sterile list of symptoms that sound all too similar, I have taken six cases from my practice and have put them into an actual life context. Set in New York City, these cases will bring you into the lives of those patients who have indeed 'slipped through the cracks'. Obviously, I have taken some creative license in producing a fictional, anonymized narrative of their experience of illness. This form is what I have designated as the 'creative medical case narrative', similar to a minimal short story.

It is my hope that you will engage empathetically with each narrative. The term 'empathy', comes from the German '*einfuhlung*', which literally means 'in-feeling', or 'feeling into'.

Pay attention to the impact of tick-borne disease on each individual's unique life. Whether it be a retired schoolteacher or a pre-adolescent boy, each individual responds to his or her diagnosis differently. Each patient experiences differently the frustration and humiliation of visiting multiple specialists, undergoing inadequate treatment and suffering persistent infection, even social rejection. Yet, nonetheless, 'similarities and commonalities' that transcend age, cultural or environmental differences emerge.

Raw case materials have their place in medical conferences and scientific journals, and they are critical in understanding the clinical realities of a disease syndrome such as Lyme disease. I am attempting to do something different as a psychiatrist/tick-borne disease physician. I wish to make the illness more personal and 'upfront' for the reader. These medical narratives illustrate themes, common symptoms and almost identical experiences that unify rather than separate them. The reader must look for what unifies them, and, if necessary, relate them to his/her own situation. For those who intuit that they are already lost in this maze of Lyme disease, my hope is that you can learn how to navigate it from this book.

However, before we move on to the narratives I have included a short chapter giving basic information about tick-borne diseases and the organisms that cause them. This section should allow our readers to gain the basic knowledge needed about Lyme and tick-borne disease, to dive into more complex case analysis.

Chapter 4

Tick-borne disease – the basics

In order to understand the themes, concepts, and discussions throughout this book, it is important to first secure a solid understanding of the basics of Lyme disease and the associated tick-borne diseases (TBDs). Throughout this book, you will hear from many experts around the world about the state of Lyme disease and TBD in their home countries. It is important to me that this book holds the voices and perspectives of many physicians, scientists, patients, and experts, as I feel that conversations about Lyme and TBD are often held in silos. One voice will not change this course of this epidemic, but many can.

My colleague, Douglas W. Fearn, has authored seven editions of a plain-language introduction to TBD, published annually by The Lyme Disease Association of Southeastern Pennsylvania, Inc. His most recent edition of this booklet, published in April of 2017, is one of the strongest overviews of the basics of Lyme disease that I have read in my career. He has kindly offered to share excerpts of his frequently asked questions with us, which I have included below.

Before we go on, we'd like briefly to introduce the life cycle of the tick and the moment that the spirochete *Borrelia burgdorferi* is introduced into that life cycle, as this has implications for the spread of Lyme disease and the increasing rates of infection around the world. The life cycle of the spirochete relates to the life cycle of specific tick species, which over two years go through four stages: egg, larva, nymph and adult – see Figure 1 below. At each stage the tick needs a blood meal in order to mature. The tick normally acquires the spirochete (Borrelia) at the larval stage when it feeds on small animals such as mice or birds, especially the white-footed mouse in the US. Though most people assume deer are the primary vector for Lyme, these smaller animals are also serious culprits. The tick then harbors the spirochete until it needs another blood meal, at which time it passes the infection on to another mammal – which could be a human.

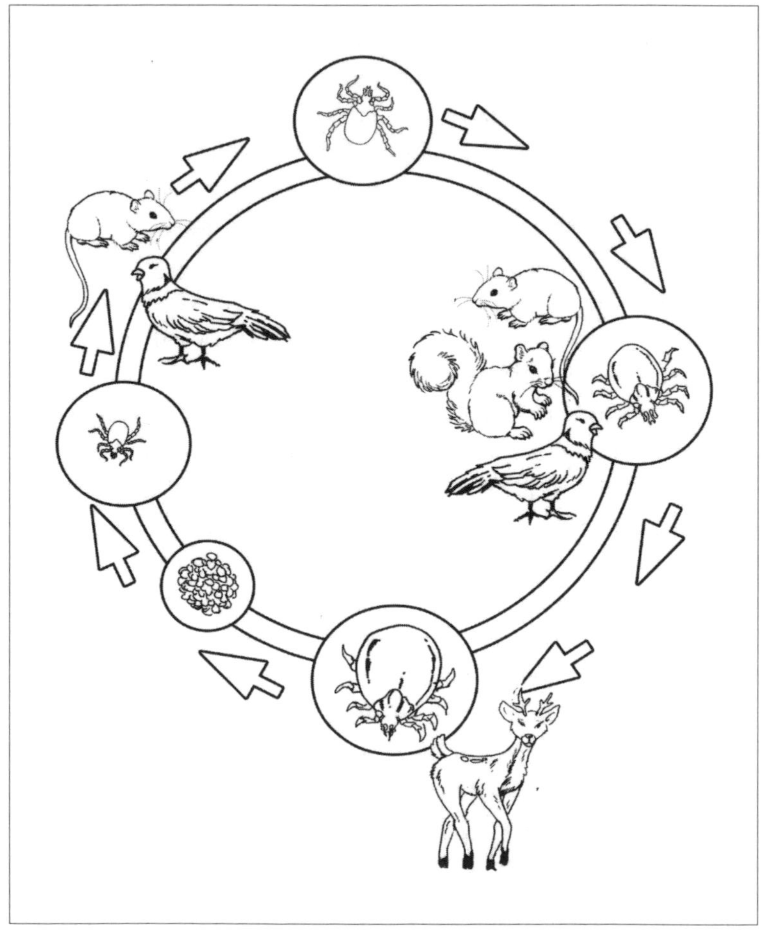

Answers to the most commonly asked questions:

By Douglas W. Fearn

Q. What is Lyme disease?

A. Lyme disease is a bacterial infection, most commonly contracted from a tick bite, that may initially cause a 'flu-like sickness. Untreated, or inadequately treated, it may cause long-term, persistent illness that can affect many systems of the body. Other tick-borne diseases are often contracted at the same time. Lyme disease is caused by a bacterial spirochete, *Borrelia burgdorferi* (Bb).

Q. How do you get it?

A. Lyme Disease (LD) is spread primarily through the bite of the deer tick, and the black-legged tick. In the US the Lone Star tick has also been associated with Lyme disease. Some researchers believe that other ticks and some other biting insects, such as mosquitoes, fleas, biting flies and lice, may also transmit LD. Babies may be born infected if the mother is infected, or possibly acquire it through breast milk. A blood transfusion with Lyme-infected blood may transmit the disease to the recipient, although this has only been proven for babesiosis, another common tick-borne disease caused by the Babesia bacterium (see below). Some medical researchers believe that Lyme, or other tick-borne diseases, can be sexually transmitted, although there has never been any research to prove that Lyme spirochetes have been found in any bodily fluids.

Q. How do I know if I have Lyme disease?

A. This can be a problem because the symptoms of LD are similar to those of many common infections, and mimic some of the symptoms of other diseases. One sign that is unmistakable is the development of a 'bullseye' rash around the site of a tick bite.

If you have this rash, you have Lyme disease. The Lyme rash varies considerably in different people, but it is typically centered on the tick bite and may range from a fraction of an inch to many inches in diameter. It may be colored anywhere from a mild red to a deep purple. It may appear a few days or even several weeks after the bite. Two weeks is typical. It may spread to other areas of the body, or there may be additional rashes, which may be far from the primary one. The classic rash has concentric areas of lighter and darker colors and expands with time, but the rash is not always in a bullseye form. It is usually painless, but it may be warm to the touch and may itch. Typically, it is flat, but some people have raised areas or bumps in the rash. Unfortunately, not everyone develops a rash, and many people fail to notice it if it is in a hard-to-see location, such as the scalp. Fewer than half the people who develop LD recall a rash or a tick bite. Other symptoms may appear at the same time. These often mimic a cold or 'flu, with fever, headache, muscle and joint pains, and/or general fatigue, but usually without nasal congestion. Early Lyme can produce a wide range of symptoms, or no symptoms at all, and is different in each person. The varied symptoms may change rapidly, sometimes within hours. The symptoms may disappear in a few days or weeks (even without treatment), or may be so minor that the infected person barely notices them. Since the 'flu season is during the winter months, and most LD infections occur during the summer, any case of "flu' in summertime should be considered suspect.

Q. How long does the disease last?

A. Even if these initial symptoms subside, the bacteria can remain in your body and may harm you later. In other cases, symptoms become increasingly severe, requiring prompt medical attention. In persistent Lyme disease, the most frequent symptoms are severe fatigue, pains that seem to have no obvious cause, and neurological and/or psychiatric problems. The disease may involve multiple body systems and organs. Symptoms may be complicated by other tick-borne co-infections acquired from the same or another tick bite. Doctors with experience in treating Lyme disease often prescribe no less than six weeks of antibiotic treatment for a tick bite with a bullseye rash. If your doctor does not agree with this approach, it may be prudent to search for a doctor who will support extended treatment. Short-term treatment has been associated with a greater likelihood of relapse.

Q. Is there a test for LD?

A. According to many experts, there is no reliable test for Lyme disease at this time. Your doctor should base his or her diagnosis on your symptoms, medical history, and your exposure to ticks. Doctors should not rely solely on tests. There are several blood tests available, but all have limitations. The blood test typically used by most family doctors, called an ELISA (or Lyme titer) test, means nothing if it is negative, and it rarely indicates infection if it is performed too early (two to six weeks after the tick bite) because your immune system has not yet made the antibodies the test is looking for. Medical experts emphasize that LD requires a clinical diagnosis, which means that the doctor should examine the patient for typical LD signs, listen to the patient's history and description of his or her symptoms and use this information to make a determination. Blood tests are usually done at the same time, but should not be relied upon. According to ILADS (the International Lyme and Associated Diseases Society), if the doctor suspects LD, and sees little reason to believe the patient has some other disease, he or she should begin antibiotic treatment without delay. Of course, doctors should also perform general blood and other tests to rule out other diseases or conditions.

Q. How many cases of Lyme disease are there really?

A. No one really knows. Some studies indicate that perhaps only one in 75 cases in the US gets into the CDC official statistics. It could be even fewer than that. Many US state health departments have decided to process only a portion of the reports, and other states have stopped reporting altogether. We do know that the actual number of cases is far, far higher than the 30,000 per year that appear in the CDC statistics. Research by the CDC in 2014 indicated that the actual number is between 300,000 and 420,000 annually in the US.

Q. What are the 'co-infections' and 'associated diseases'?

A. The ticks that carry the Lyme bacteria also often carry other micro-organisms that cause other diseases. The most common 'co-infections' are anaplasmosis, ehrlichiosis, babesiosis, bartonellosis and Rocky Mountain spotted fever. Anaplasmosis, ehrlichiosis and Rocky Mountain spotted fever may be cured by the same antibiotics that are prescribed for Lyme disease. New tick-borne diseases are being discovered all the time, and some established diseases are being diagnosed more often. Our knowledge continues to grow.

Co-infections: the horsemen of the apocalypse

Bartonella

It is difficult to imagine that after Borrelia was discovered in 1982 and became the infamous Lyme disease spirochete, other pathogens harbored in the tick gut remained unknown, and yet could cause serious disease – a sobering thought, since it was generally believed that modern medicine had uncovered almost all of the common bacterial pathogens that regularly cause human disease. Then along came **Bartonella**. An excellent paper in the *Journal of Pediatrics* May 2008 issue, entitled 'Beyond Cat Scratch Disease. Widening the Spectrum of *Bartonella henselae*' and authored by Todd A. Florin MD et al. from the University of Pennsylvania, explained that CSD (cat scratch disease) was described over 50 years ago and it was only a little more than a scant 25 years ago that the actual Bartonella organism was identified, in 1983. Wear et al discovered a small, aerobic, pleomorphic gram-negative bacillus in infected lymph nodes of patients with CSD. In 1991 it was finally isolated and cultured. Today the genus Bartonella includes 19 different species of which a minimum of six are responsible for human disease. These are *B. henselae, B. baciliformis, B. quintana, B. elizabethae, B. vinsonii* and *B. koehlerae*. In infected patients the organisms are found most commonly in blood vessel walls (intracellular endothelial cells and erythrocyte organisms seen in clumps inside the cell). They are also seen in macrophages (white blood cells) lining the sinuses of lymph nodes, in nodal germinal centers, in non-necrotic areas of inflammation and in areas of suppurating necrosis. Since they are also intraerythrocytic parasites, they evade the host immune response, which makes blood immune testing very difficult, with only 20-25 per cent positive results in clinically infected patients. For individuals with an intact immune system, the infection remains primarily within the lymphatics with a symptomatic immune response that can last anywhere from two months to two years in chronic cases. In a paper by Adelson et al (2004) looking at infections carried by ticks in New Jersey the authors found that 34.5 per cent of the ticks analyzed by PCR technology carried Bartonella.[25] Here we have a newcomer bacterium emerging from obscurity. A little more than 20 years after the discovery of *Borrelia burgdorferi*, living in the same tick abdomen, a new virulent pathogen is uncovered. Remarkable! The discovery of this new intracellular pathogen changes the 'one bacterium' paradigm. The physician must now consider a 'co-infection synergy' causing the complex symptom presentation of the tick-infected patient. The consequences of this new major discovery are far reaching in their clinical importance. It dramatically changes the face of TBD and exponentially complicates diagnosis and treatment.

An interesting characteristic pertaining to Bartonella is that it adheres to, or is phagocytosed (engulfed), by macrophages. These cells secrete 'vascular endothelial growth factor' (VEGF). VEGF is thought to act as an endothelial wall inducer leading to the proliferation of endothelial cells and angiogenesis (the development of new blood vessels). On testing, a high level of VEGF is an indication that the individual may be harboring the bacterium. Cats used to be the main reservoir of this bacterium and the seropositive prevalence in cats in the hot humid US states was found to be as high as 51 per cent. The bacterium was found to be transported by the insect vector, the 'cat flea' or *Clenocephalides felis*. It has recently been found also in dogs (in 27 per cent of sick dogs in the southeast US). It was a scant 15 years ago that it was determined that the *Ixodes scapularis* tick was also a carrier of this Bartonella bacteria. It follows logically, that it must be considered as one of the important co-infections along with Babesia also transmitted by the tick.

It strikes me as incredible that this organism lay undiscovered for all of medical history, until it was finally uncovered as a serious source of illness in the 1980s, first as the cause of CSD transmitted by its flea insect vector; then in the early 2000s it was proven to be transported by the tick, *Ixodes scapularis*. Even today in 2019 there is debate and skepticism as to whether the disease can be transferred by the bite of a tick. Incredibly, there are still 'minds' that are rigidly locked onto a single hypothesis. These physicians refuse to consider new published science that disputes their old mind set.

Manifestations and symptoms of bartonellosis

1. Fever of unknown origin (FUO)
2. Liver and spleen problems ('hepatosplenic presentation') – There can be microabscesses in the liver and spleen, usually diagnosed with the help of abdominal imaging (CAT scan). Often there is exquisite abdominal pain, which can be crippling.

3. Loss of appetite with weight loss – Gastroparesis with difficulty digesting food and major food allergies (corn, gluten, dairy, sugar, etc)
4. Anorexia or bulimia
5. Intermittent nausea throughout the day with no apparent precipitant like a meal
6. Headache described as gripping the head in a vice evolving into full-blown migraine
7. Ocular symptoms – Blurred vision, pain behind the eyes (pressure or stabbing), sudden change of glasses prescription, dry eyes with inflamed tear ducts, uveitis, optic neuritis, neuroretinits, abnormal color vision
8. Pain in the bottoms of the feet – Feels like walking on broken glass, particularly in the morning
9. Sudden psychiatric manifestions – Extreme anxiety, depression, mania, negative thought intrusion (suicidal thoughts, sudden urges to hurt a loved one, paranoia, rage response out of character with individual's character), over the top for little or no reason
10. Excessive sensitivity to light and sound – Unable to tolerate florescent lights; noises like ice clinking in a glass, or a person chewing food cause high irritablity
11. Weird nightmarish dreams, often of dismemberment, vampires sucking blood etc
12. Insomnia with poor sleep quality
13. Rashes including stria (red strips often on abdomen, axilla, back), angiomata, easy bruising, lesions without any known trauma, tender lumps and nodules along the side of the leg
14. Heart palpitations and strange chest pain
15. Recurring sore throats
16. Peripheral neuropathies or nerve irritation (burning, vibrating, numb, shooting, electric shock type nerve pain but with normal EMG results)
17. Ringing in the ears (tinnitus) and hearing problems

18. Tremors and muscle twitching
19. Episodes of confusion and disorientation as well as depersonalization
20. Swollen lymph nodes, especially under the arms and in the neck and groin
21. Sticky or thick sweat, often in the morning or late afternoon
22. Stroke.

Diagnosis of bartonellosis

Once again, because of the nature of the infection with Bartonella, the serological diagnosis is very difficult and can be misleading for the clinician. Isolation in cultures is difficult, requiring a two to six week incubation period for primary isolation, with less than 50 per cent success. PCR (polymerase chain reaction) has been almost 100 per cent specific but lacks sensitivity (less than 40 per cent in one study). It also needs highly specialized equipment and trained personnel. Two main serological tests are currently in use: IFA (indirect immunoflorescent assay) and EIA (enzyme immune assay). Positive IgM EIA, as in Lyme disease, indicates active disease. The duration of IgM antibodies that can be detected lasts less than three months. The problem for clinicians who suspect Bartonella has been this short duration of IgM antibodies. Once again, as in Lyme disease, the same stubborn irritating fact prevails: a negative test does exclude *acute* disease. And since the Bartonella bacterium is intracellular – inside endothelial walls, erythrocytes and macrophages – it is even more elusive, giving few serological clues to its existence. After all, it took bacteriological science and infectious disease medicine until 1985 to discover the fact that 29 different subtypes of Bartonella existed, with six of them being pathogens. Worse, on testing IgG EIA after one year, less than 25 per cent continue to show positive seriology. It then becomes increasingly difficult to diagnose an active infection from a previous infection. Once again, there is the slippery slope when relying on making a diagnosis through blood testing only. Ultimately, like borreliosis, bartonellosis is still strictly a clinical diagnosis.

Treatment for bartonellosis

The treatment of Bartonella infection is dependent on the clinical manifestations, the immune status of the patient and the number of co-infections the patient is suffering from. Unfortunately, as in the case of borreliosis, there is minimal data in the literature as to the most effective treatment for this organism. Randomized controlled trials are few. The published 'in vitro' (laboratory) studies show susceptibility to many classes of antibiotics: macrolides, beta-lactams, cephalsporins, bactrin, rifampin, rifabutin, quinolone and aminoglycosides (gentamicin). Sadly, the 'in vitro' studies have not been replicated 'in vivo' clinically in humans. Most of the antibiotics mentioned showed bacteriostatic activity. Only the aminoglycosides showed bactericidal activity. Lack of cell membrane penetration, the intracellularity of the organisms spread out through the patient's system, the fact that its habitat is the vascular wall of the blood vessels, particularly the capillary bed, make it a demon to track and eliminate. In cases of encephalopathy arising from Bartonella, as well as optic retinitis and severe psychiatric disturbances, the minimum length of treatment should be no less than three months orally.

The obvious question always arises in the minds of conscientious physicians. If you can't rely on serological testing and the clinical picture is all mixed together like an alphabet soup, then: 'How the hell does one diagnose and treat the damn bug?' How, indeed! Some clinical clues may help the befuddled doc. The group of symptoms listed above appear regularly in my practice, and are tell-tale clues to Bartonella co-infection.

Babesia

It's a challenge to the clinician that s/he has to deal with two extremely difficult micro-organisms like Borrellia and

Bartonella. Their symptoms can often overlap to create an extremely complicated symptom complex with important diagnostic implications for the patient. However, to muddy the waters even further, a third organism – Babesia – is also a common co-infection; it pirates a patient's red blood cells and causes serious immune complications and oxygen deprivation of tissues. The first reference in the literature to this stealth parasite is in the Bible (Exodus 9.3): when the then Pharaoh would not allow the Israelites to leave Egypt, God visited a deadly plague onto the Egyptians' livestock and all their animals died in the field.

In 1988, Victor Babes MD (after whom the microbe is named) published a paper identifying the organism as an intracellular erythrocyte (red blood cell) parasite of domesticated animals. Over the last 50 years, *Babesia app.* has been increasingly identified as causing serious infection, not only in livestock but also in humans. The first human case of Babesia was identified in 1957 in Croatia. A farmer who had been working in tick-infested pastures presented with fever, anemia and hemoglobinuria, and died two weeks later.

Then Smith and Kilborne, working in the US, identified a similar organism in Texas cattle. A cattle tick (*Boophilius annulatis*) was found to be capable of transmitting the infectious parasite to vertebrate hosts. More than 100 species of babesiosis have been identified since then in wild and domestic animals and humans.

Closer to home, I personally have treated well over 50 patients in my practice who have vacationed on Cape Cod, Massachusetts (particularly on the Island of Nantucket, as well as Block Island, Rhode Island) who have been infected with Babesia. The East coast of the US, including the states of Massachusetts, Rhode Island, New York, Connecticut, Maine and Vermont have become endemic areas for babesiosis.

The discerning physician must be aware of the strong possibility that there are a minimum of three pathogens that need to be diagnosed and treated in a TBD patient. Other pathogens, such as *Rickettsia rickettsiae*, granulocytic Anaplasma, *Mycoplasma fermentans* and numerous viruses, must also be considered as contributing to the overall illness of the compromised patient. It is not the purpose of this book, however, to delve into all the possible co-infection combinations. In my practice the three debilitating 'Bs', Borrelia, Bartonella, and Babesia, make up a good 80 per cent of TBD combinations that I treat.

The commonest species in North America to infect humans is *Babesia microti* and it is transmitted by the same tick as Borrellia – namely, *Ixodes scapularis*. The primary reservoir is the same as Borrelia, the white-footed mouse. In areas where there is greater biodiversity, other vertebrate mammals can also be reservoir hosts (moles, chipmunks, squirrels, possums, foxes, as well as birds). The parasitic pathogen comes from the same phylum (family) as malaria (Plasmodium), Toxoplasma and Cryptosporidium.

Babesia, like malaria, has a complicated life cycle which involves 'asexual reproduction' in the erythrocytes of their mammalian hosts, but 'sexual reproduction' in the ticks. The morphology (structure) of the organism at each stage is given a different name: trophozoites (which are inside red blood cells and divide by budding), merozoites (which invade other red cells), gametocytes (ingested by the tick along with the blood), ookinetes (which invade the tick's salivary glands) and sporoblasts (which remain dormant while the engorged tick sheds its outer skin). At the next tick blood meal, sporoblasts are activated and can liberate up to 10,000 sporozoites, which enter the salivary glands of the tick and then directly invade the vertebrate host via the skin. All active tick stages feed on the white-tailed deer which is an important host for the tick, but not a reservoir for *Babesia microti*. However, the deer serve to amplify the number of ticks, hence the increase in human cases.

Nature produces a complex two-year ballet of a 'tick-host life cycle' coordinated over the same period with the life cycle of the Babesiosis parasite. This dance is amazingly intertwined and timed exquisitely to support the survival of both species!

Clinical manifestations of babesiosis

The more academic understanding of the presentation of babesiosis divides its signs and symptoms into three categories: (i) mild to moderate viral-like illness; (ii) severe disease, especially in patients with poor spleen function in whom it can lead to death; (iii) asymptomatic illness. The symptoms include: gradual onset of malaise and fatigue, followed by fever, chills, sweats, headache, arthralgia , myalgia and anorexia. Unfortunately, a great number of these symptoms blend into bartonellosis and borreliosis.

In my practice, there are eight 'red flags' that help separate out babesiosis from the two others:

1. Crushing fatigue morphing into exhaustion: The patient is mostly bedridden and the slightest expenditure of energy cause profound debilitating exhaustion. As one 22-year-old female college student stated: 'When it's bad, I can hardly get out of bed. Just to go to the bathroom requires an enormous amount of energy. I can't plan anything, because if I do manage to get out of the house, I'm so wiped by the end of the event that I need two or three days to recover. I can sleep 18 hours a day and not feel rested. I go from the bed to the couch and back to the bed again. I never make any plans to go out with my friends because I never know if I will have the energy to do anything at all. I've been diagnosed with Epstein Barr virus, chronic fatigue, depression and hypothyroidism and tried all kinds of medications and vitamins; nothing helps. I feel like my body has completely run out of gas. I used be a cross-country runner for my high school; now I'm lucky if I can go from the couch to the bathroom without getting winded!'
2. Shortness of breath and/or air hunger: Patients complain classically that they are winded going up stairs. One patient, a 42-year-old advertising executive, said: 'I feel older than my 72-year-old father. I'm always tired and

I can hardly get up the stairs to my walkup on the third floor without having to stop and rest two or three times. I don't go to the gym anymore. I feel terrible after the workout. I've become a slug.'

3. Drenching night sweats: The Babesia patient will invariably experience temperature regulation issues which result in drenching night sweats and excessive perspiration during the day. One patient, a 50-year-old housewife, stated: 'I know it's not menopause, I've been through that "delightful" phase almost seven years ago. This is different. Before it was sudden, hot, uncontrollable flashes, but minimal sweating. At night I wake up in a pool of perspiration. I have to change everything. Nightgown, sheets, everything. Now I keep an extra nightgown by the bed, two of my large beach towels and an extra set of sheets. My poor husband, he's so patient! He tells me that he's going to buy us flotation cushions to save us both from drowning. And I can't seem to get comfortable with temperature. I'm either opening or closing the windows or turning off and on the air conditioner, and as soon as I take a shower, dry myself off and dress, I'm perspiring again. It's driving me crazy!'
4. Myalgia: The patient complains of persistent muscle soreness. 'It's like I've run a marathon twice over,' said one male patient, a 36-year-old fireman. 'I used to be in pretty good shape. You kind of have to be if you are doing my job. But this is ridiculous. It's not my joints so much; they're okay. It's my muscles. They're always as sore as hell. I take hot showers, go to the spa, get my wife to massage my legs and arms, use lidocaine patches, take naprosyn, go to the chiropractor for adjustment. Nothing helps. The muscles remain sore as hell. The pain just doesn't go away.'
5. Headaches: The patient can suddenly acquire persistent pounding headaches that can often evolve into migraine-type severe episodes. A 17-year-old teenage boy stated:

'I was never a headache person. My older sister was always having headaches with her period. I thought to myself what a bum deal to have to go through this every month. I was glad I wasn't a girl. Now I understand how she must have been suffering. I've been getting these pounding headaches regularly. It's like someone is beating a drum on the inside of my temples. Nothing takes it away except migraine medication, and that doesn't even work all the time. And I can't take it every day. I can go to bed with the headache, sleep the night through, and wake up with the same pounding headache. I've already tried a lot of different medications, even botox injections. Nothing takes them away.'

6. Weight gain: Patients complain that weight gain started after a 'flu like illness with fever, and it continued for no apparent reason. One patient recounted this incident. 'I'm beside myself. Look at me. After the 'flu the summer we came back from the Cape, I began to put on weight for no reason at all. I have gained more then 30 lb over the last two years. I just can't get it off. I've tried every diet imaginable and then some. I've starved myself for weeks and I don't lose more than two pounds. Diuretics do nothing, just make me urinate more, that's all. I try to work out. I've hired a trainer for when I go to the gym three times per week. It takes everything out of me, but I push through it. I can't stand this weight. Nothing in my wardrobe fits. I refuse to buy bigger sizes. I'm miserable!'
7. Pathogenesis: What makes babesiosis such a difficult disease for my patients are two major processes: 'erythrocyte modification' by the pathogen and the 'host immune response' to the pathogen. When the merozoites leave an infected red blood cell (erythrocyte) there is loss of cell membrane integrity, with eventual destruction of the erythrocyte and the development of hemolytic anemia and tissue hypoxia. In addition, there is cytoadherence

leading to microvascular obstruction and tissue hypoxia, especially in the large muscle masses which need increased blood flow to oxygenate the tissue.

8. Immunologically TNF-alpha (tumor necrosis factor-alpha) along with other cytokines activate macrophages to produce nitric oxide that kills intracellular parasites. Pulmonary inflammation is the most common complication in people experiencing severe *B. microti* infection. Others show non-cardiac pulmonary edema. Immune compromised and a-splenic patients have the worst outcomes brought about by low CD4 T cell activation that can lead to fulminating and persistent parasitosis, with eventual death.

However, the clinical condition that most frequents my practice is a mixed bag of TBD bacteria and parasites. One set of symptoms belonging to one pathogen wraps around the other two like a vine growing around a tree.

Diagnosis of Babesia infestation

Again, as in Lyme disease and Bartonella, we are forced to make a clinical diagnosis. We have sophisticated tests for babesiosis, such as microscopic examination of slides for evidence of parasitic infestation of erythrocytes, IgG and IgM antibody assessment, PCR for DNA, Tick-plex nanotechnology, gamma-interferon measurement, T-cell stimulation with spirochetes, and the ELISA peptide immune assay. Unfortunately, the tests are not reliable enough to make a diagnosis or follow a treatment course most of the time. Only the symptom recognition and quality of improvement can tell the real story. Frustratingly, like borreliosis, a negative test does not rule out an active infection.

Treatment for babesiosis

Treatment can be long and complicated as the physician is dealing with a minimum of three completely different pathogens at the same time (and probably more). The subtleties of treatment are not the focus of this book. Suffice it to say, it is often like walking a tightrope with a patient. The following medications are used in different combinations with different patients, depending of course on their symptoms, how they react to the medication and the strength of their immune system:

Coartem (anti malarial)
Mepron (anti pneumocystis carnii)
Zithromax (macrolide intracellular)
Bactrin DS (sulfa drug)
Alinia (cryptosporidium)
Dapsone, (leprosy)
Pyrazinamide (antiparasitic)
Doxy or minocycline.

I usually treat with some combination of these medications for at least six months. Other auxiliary treatments include hyperbaric O2, ozone infusions and blood replacement with red cell transfusion.

There is an interesting viewpoint offered by Hope McIntyre MD, a physician member of ILADS, in an unpublished paper written in 2013. She suggests a number of insights.

1. Babesiosis causes false positive Lyme disease testing by producing cross reactive antibodies due to activation of B cells.
2. Most babesiosis is resistant to the standard treatment of Mepron and Zithromax. They suppress the symptoms, but the patient relapses when they are stopped.
3. Babesiosis antibodies don't develop until after the patient has cleared the infection. The sicker the patient, the fewer the antibodies they will make. Once the infection is cleared the antibody titres will rise, ironically provding proof that in fact the patient had the disease.
4. Standard labs render blood smears for babesiosis

completely worthless. If venous blood is used, the slide needs to be prepared and viewed within an hour of the blood draw, otherwise the morphology changes and the parasites will not be seen.

5. Babesiosis is a public health crisis, especially in endemic areas, because of the possibility of a tainted blood supply coming from unsuspecting donors.
6. Babesiosis is the underlying cause of many serious chronic diseases. Hyper coagulability (blood clots too easily) is one of the underlying mechanism, as is small vessel vasculitis. The list is extensive. Among some of the diseases implicated: ALS (motor neurone disease), Alzheimer's dementia, aneurysms, anxiety disorders, autism and autism-spectrum disorder, bipolar disorder, chronic fatigue syndrome, depression, ITP, inflammatory bowel disease, failing memory, neurocognitve disability, food sensitivities and interstitial cystitis.

All of these diseases and many more are on her list of possible diseases enabled by or directly aided by babesiosis. A compelling hypothesis to say the least!

Rickettsia rickettsia

Rickettsia rickettsia, originally named 'the black measles' because of its spotted rash appearance throughout the body, fortunately has not shown itself in my office over the past 35 years. Therefore, I have no clinical experience with this organism. Its importance is unmistakable, however. It is found around the world on every continent (except Antarctica). It tends to thrive in warm damp places. It is a gram-negative intracellular coccobacillus bacteria from the class 'alphaproteobacteria' which causes Rocky Mountain spotted fever. It is one of the more pathogenic rickettsial strains, found mostly in the Western mountain US states. It was discovered by Howard Ricketts of the University of Chicago in 1902; at that time the infection had an 80-90 per cent mortality rate. Ricketts was a fearless, committed scientist who, to further his research on this organism (remember, this was a time of no antibiotics), injected himself with various pathogens to measure their effects on his system. Tragically he died at the age 41, in all likelihood from an infectious agent from his laboratory.

Wolbach gave the first detailed description of this pathogen, recognizing it as an intracellular bacterium found in endothelial cells.

The organism is carried in the same tick, *Ixodes scapularis,* as the three Bs. In this case, unlike the other three microorganisms, ticks can be vectors, reservoirs and amplifiers of this disease all at the same time. An uninfected tick can be infected by feeding on an infected 'vertebrate' host. During the larval or nymph stage, the mode of transmission is called 'transstadial transmission'. Once the tick becomes infected, it will be infected for life! An infected male tick can transmit the bacterium to an unaffected female, who in turn can transmit the infection to offspring, a mechanism known as 'transovarian passage'. The bacterium can then be transmitted to mammals through infected tick feces coming into contact with an open wound or eating food that contains tick feces. Of course, the most likely transmission to humans is through the bite of an infected tick. A fascinating fact concerning the Rickettsia bacterium is that it can eradicate 'males' and undergo parthenogenesis (reproduction without fertilization). By eradicating male hosts, the female host can pass the *R. rickettsia* gene to her offspring. This is another method of survival and another way to infect a mammalian host.

It has evolved a number of mechanisms or 'virulence' factors to invade the immune system and thus infect humans. The bacterium enters the endothelial cells and alters their 'cytoskeleton', which in turn induces phagocytosis (cell death). Now the gene can be replicated and further invade other cells in the body.

Clinical presentation:

Once again, we are faced with the same dilemma as with the three Bs. *R. rickettsia* infection is a clinical diagnosis based on history, endemic area and tick exposure as well as signs and symptoms of the disease. Laboratory identification confirms the diagnosis. Unfortunately, onset of the condition can be non-specific. The early symptoms usually include fever, GI symptoms (nausea, vomiting, abdominal pain, loss of appetite), malaise, myalgia, conjunctivitis (red eyes), photophobia, cranial or motor nerve paralysis, sudden transient deafness, and maculopapular rash two to five days after the onset of fever, usually appearing first on the forearms, wrists and ankles, and sometimes the palms and the soles.

Ten per cent of those infected never develop a rash at all. Petechial rash (pin-head brown or red spots) is considered a sign of progression to severe disease. Antibodies to *R. rickettsia* are detectable seven to 10 days after the illness begins. Treatment should be started immediately if the infection is suspected because if it is initiated too late, serious complications can occur in cardiovascular, respiratory, CNS, gut and renal systems. This can be accompanied by thrombocytopenia, hyponatremia, septic shock, kidney failure, heart failure and death.

On an evolutionary note, 'symbiogenesis' is a theory of the origin of 'eukaryotic cells from prokaryotic' (simpler, with no nucleus) organisms. It holds that the organelles that distinguish the internal anatomy of our cellular make-up evolved through symbiosis of individual single-celled bacteria and archae (another type of prokaryotic organism). The theory holds that mitochondria, plastids such as chloroplasts, and quite possibly other organelles represent formerly free-living bacteria taken one inside the other in 'endosymbiosis'.

In more detail, the mitochondria (our cells' 'power stations') appear to be related to 'Rickettsia protobacteria' and chloroplasts to nitrogen-fixing filamentous 'cyanobacteria'. Amazing. Our disease carriers in modern times were possibly responsible for evolving complex cellular life as we know it today in living creatures millions of years ago!

Anaplasmosis

This organism was formerly known as HGE (human granulocytic Ehrlichiosis) and was only recently detected in 1994. It has the same distribution in the upper mid-west and the northeast of the US as Borrelia and similarly follows the same distribution in Europe as Borrelia. The organism that causes the disease is known as *Anaplasma phagocytophilum*. It is difficult to diagnose because the symptoms blend in with the four other bacteria already discussed, Borrelia, Babesia, Bartonella and Rickettsia – namely, fatigue, fever and chills. However, the complications of this seemingly innocuous disease can be life threatening depending on the age and general health of the patient infected. One article quoted a figure of 50 per cent or more of patients who were symptomatic of the illness being hospitalized. After a tick bite, the acute and dangerous tell-tale sign is a high fever over 103°F (39.4°C). The chronic tell-tale sign is increased susceptibility to infection. In a Borrelia endemic area, this is an important clue to the possibility of this disease. This illness can be especially problematic in children if antibiotic treatment is not started immediately. It can lead to excruciating headaches, GI symptoms, stiff neck, confusion, hemorrhages and renal failure.

Pathogenesis – how anaplasmosis develops

In a paper entitled 'Breaking in and Grabbing a Meal: *Anaplasma phagocytophilum* cellular invasion, nutrient acquisition and promising tools for their study' the authors, Hily Truchan and colleagues, describe intricate mechanisms for the pathogen's survival. The bacterium expresses its pathology by invading white cells (granulocytes), bone marrow and endothelial cells. Since the white cells are critical in first-line immunological response to bacteria, the invasion by this obligatory intracellular parasite contributes to the human host's vulnerability to other infections.

Anaplasma has invasin-host cell receptor interactions. As a result this promotes bacterial entry and the degradation, as well as diversion, of cell membrane traffic pathways. The organism cleverly exploits these pathways to route essential nutrients to the host organelle (a vacuole). It resides in this protective niche, which it remodels for its own survival purposes. The organism re-routes the host's cell membrane traffic, which allows for the transfer and delivery of vital nutrients to the bacterium. This process, which includes attachment and entry into the host cell, is facilitated by multiple bacterial adhesins / invasins. The bacterium also stabilizes its own outer membrane by incorporating cholesterol which it hijacks from its mammalian host. Not only is exogenous cholesterol taken up by the bacterium, but endogenous cholesterol synthesis is up-regulated. This suggests that cholesterol plays an important role in the virulence of the *A. phagocytophilium*. The dependence on cholesterol indicates that patients, especially older patients with hypercholesterolemia, may experience more severe infections. Dietary changes, such as a low cholesterol diet, may be helpful in aiding the control of the infection. In my practice, almost without exception, the Paleo type of nutritional protocol is highly recommended.

Diagnosis of anaplasmosis

As usual, the physician is forced to make a clinical diagnosis. Antibody studies can be unhelpful and often times negative. Elevated IgM antibodies are less specific than IgG and cause cross reactions leading to false positive tests. PCR for DNA is specific but not sensitive. So unhappily (as with all the bacteria and parasites that the tick transfers to humans), it can discharge a bellyful of pathogens into its human host that elude sophisticated laboratory validation of their presence. More clues can be found in a lowered white cell count, elevated liver enzymes, mild anemia and thrombocytopenia (lowered platelet count).

Treatment for anaplasmosis

Fortunately, the treatment for anaplasmosis is for the most part the same as for borreliosis. The antibiotics doxycycline, azithromycin and ceftin all appear effective. With a low white cell count, although a suggestive marker for this disease, one has to be aware of the possibility of viral transmission (EBV, CMV, HHV6).

Part Two

The intuitive clinical case narratives

Chapter 5

Alex Peterson, age 8 years
The trouble with diagnosis

The Peterson family were diehard Upper West Siders. They enjoyed all the advantages of living close to Lincoln Center and some of the best restaurants in the city. Though they had enjoyed their three weeks alone together over the summer, they were looking forward to picking up their son, Alex, in the Berkshires. He'd been there two successive summers, and loved the camp because of its emphasis on the outdoors. He particularly enjoyed the three-night camp-outs in tents under the stars. In the middle of the night, he'd sneak out of his sleeping bag and just gaze at the wondrous sky. Every summer, he would get the odd mosquito bite here or there, and once even a spider bite that left a red mark, but it went away after a few days, leaving nothing but a small red spot on his thigh. By the end of camp, he'd forgotten about it.

When the Petersons came to pick Alex up that summer, he wasn't his usual self. He appeared subdued and cranky. When he arrived back home, he preferred to stay in his room and play video games, or sit on the sofa in the family room and watch TV.

Two weeks before school started, Alex suddenly claimed that most of his muscles and joints were hurting, that his neck was killing him, and he was always feeling hot and sweaty, especially at night. A couple of times he had soaked right through his sheets. His nights were unusually restless. Usually he slept like a log the moment his head hit the pillow, but over the previous two weeks he had been jerking and twisting in his sleep, waking frequently.

It was impossible to get him up in the morning. He seemed dead to the world. His mother could hardly wake him.

When school started, his low energy and fatigue did not get better. For the first time since he had started school, he had six late marks and five missed days on his report card in the first quarter. He slipped from an A-grade student down to a B-grade student. This had never happened before in his school career. He appeared to have no interest in his homework assignments. Often, they were left uncompleted or not handed in at all. It seemed to him that everything he did learn, he forgot just as quickly. He told his father tearfully one evening when they were alone, and he had brought back a C-grade in math, that numbers were now very confusing to him. Moreover, he couldn't concentrate on anything, not even his favorite video games. Perhaps it was because he was so physically uncomfortable, or because school had become such a problem, but it was clear to everyone – parents, teachers, friends, and even his kid sister, Jackie – that his personality had changed drastically. He had gone from a well-adjusted, open, friendly, socially active, sports-minded kid to a morose, irritable, low energy, difficult and angry child.

Alex had at least two pediatrician visits with Dr Hardy in just six weeks. He had been a patient of this concerned and friendly doctor since birth. Dr Hardy knew Alex extremely well and he was not an alarmist, but he was perplexed at the obvious changes in Alex's health. Significant blood testing was undertaken. X-rays of his knee, hip and vertebral joints were done, a CAT scan of his abdomen, and even an ELISA Lyme test. Dr Hardy left no stone unturned. He was exceptionally thorough. Nevertheless, all testing proved to be negative, except an Epstein Barr virus (cause of 'mono' or 'glandular fever') antibody test which was positive for IgG, which meant past exposure at some point to the virus. Dr Hardy postulated that it was probably a type of post-viral syndrome, an autoimmune-type illness that could affect muscles and joints, like the 'para virus' and cause Alex to be so fatigued. He prescribed a multivitamin and a low dose of

Focalin, a situmlant used to treat ADHD, to see if it could perk Alex up and help him focus better in school.

After a month of treatment, Alex's mother reported back to the doctor that she hadn't seen much of a change. Alex seemed a little more focused, and perhaps had a little more energy, but he seemed even more depressed. He was extremely irritable and had completely lost his appetite.

The pediatrician advised this was likely a hormonal problem. Children of Alex's age, he said, sometimes started to experience hormonal changes that were hard to adjust to. The Petersons were urged to be patient and not to panic. Growing pains could take a while. But Alex did not improve. He added more psychological symptoms to his behavior. He became severely OCD and was fixed on making sure he completed a ritualistic routine before he could get into bed and turn off the light. The rituals took at least half an hour to complete and, if interrupted for any reason, he 'd have to start all over again.

Finally, after another frantic phone call from Mrs Peterson about Alex's strange behaviors, he and his family were referred to Dr Mark Croton, a child psychiatrist on the Upper West Side with many years of experience, who taught at Columbia University. After six months with the family together, and Alex alone, Dr Croton worked his magic. Alex did in fact seem to settle down. After much discussion and trepidation, he was placed on antidepressant medication. His mood seemed to brighten, he was not as negative, and he started to do better in school. His grades improved from a C to a B and he was even playing soccer again. Alex seemed better, though definitely not back to his old self.

Three months later, Alex came down with a case of 'strep throat' that was being passed around his class. After starting amoxicillin to treat the streptococcus bacterium, Alex started to show signs of debilitating PANDAS ('pediatric autoimmune neuropsychiatric disorders associated with streptococcal infections'). It was as if all of the symptoms from the past year came roaring back in a matter of days. He stopped eating and his anxiety and OCD symptoms became out of control. He'd be up through the night, almost hyperactive, and then would be thrown into a dead sleep for hours in the day. Even the gentlest touch seemed to induce agony. The Petersons were at a complete loss for what to do.

After two full weeks of missed school, a tutor was brought in to assist Alex and try to keep him up to date with the class. Within just a few weeks, Alex's reading and math levels had dropped three grade levels. Though unsure of whether or not it was her place to step in, one afternoon the tutor asked Mrs Peterson whether or not Alex had had a neuropsychological evaluation. Had they ever considered Lyme disease? she asked. She had seen a couple of kids who had similar problems, and they too had tested negative for Lyme disease, only to find out much later that they were in fact infected with the bacterium.

Though the Petersons were excited by the idea that there might be an answer to Alex's suffering, they couldn't help but doubt the diagnosis. Alex had already been tested for Lyme disease. The results had come back negative. How could he still have this with a negative blood test? It didn't make sense, but then neither did his illness for that matter.

Relief for the family finally arrived, after yet another year of them wandering through the Lyme maze. Help came via the father of a girl who had gone to the same camp as Alex three summers prior and who had become very sick. Her symptoms sounded remarkably close to Alex's condition. She had been 'cured' by a Connecticut pediatrician and Lyme disease expert, Dr Charles Ray Jones. On researching him, Alex's family found his reputation for treating children with TBD (from infancy to 18 years) to be legendary. In his almost 60 years of dedicated medical practice, he had treated more than 10,000 children successfully for the disease.

Alex's family waited more than four months for the initial consultation with Dr Jones. They found him warm, empathic and reassuring. He put Alex's clinical history, his physical and emotional and cognitive symptoms into an understandable, medically logical, explanatory pattern. Igenex laboratory results (page 261) confirmed the diagnosis of persistent borreliosis and co-infections. Alex was treated with a nine-month course of oral and intramuscular antibiotics, and returned once again to being a healthy, normal child.

Physician analysis: the trouble with diagnosis

The Peterson case exhibits a number of 'commonalities' explored in the first section of this book (page 16). Doctors could have been alerted by:

- The sudden drastic change in Alex's personality
- The rapid change in his cognitive and intellectual abilities
- The history of his summer camp experiences, and his 'spider bites' in the highly endemic Berkshires
- The drenching night sweats, insomnia and exhaustion
- The sudden history of PANDAS.

This question about blood testing and diagnosis is yet another sticking point for patients and doctors alike around the world. Though we are starting to see impressive innovation in diagnostic testing for Lyme and tick-borne diseases, for the most part doctors are not employing these tools. Even when being admitted to some of the best hospital systems in the world, with the most cutting-edge diagnostic tools, these new diagnostic tests are simply not used. As a result, patients in many cases are not diagnosed at all.

As we stand today, the most regularly used two-tier testing approach potentially misses up to 40 per cent of infected patients. For patients who have been infected for more than 12 months, the incidence of false negative results may be well over 50 per cent.[26] ELISA assays have been found in some studies to be as high as 56 per cent false negative (depending on the kit) when compared with clinical diagnosis. Though slightly more reliable, an alternative test, the Western Blot test, is still only accurate around 80 per cent of the time. So why use these tests diagnostically? If this system is employed, one out of two patients can and will be incorrectly eliminated from treatment. Unfortunately, this system is the one most readily available to physicians around the world, and transitioning to a brand new system comes with its own flaws and hurdles. So perhaps, instead of asking why we use this test, we should be asking, why is the 'two-tier' system so flawed?

The two-tier system relies on antibody production against either the entire spirochete (*Borrelia burgdorferi*), the bacteria causing Lymed disease, or the proteins on its coat. These are numbered specifically on the Western Blot test from 18kda to 93kda.[27] 'kda' stands for kilodotan, the actual weight of the protein. The higher the number, the heaver the protein.

The CDC (Centers for Disease Control and Prevention in Atlanta, USA) needs to know how many Lyme cases occur in any given year, and in exactly what areas throughout the USA. This is known as the epidemiology of the disease. The CDC determined that a 'positive reportable test' would need to include the most frequently occurring, statistically relevant proteins. When they originally started recording this data, the CDC picked three proteins to be designated as 'statistically relevant'. The other proteins, nine in all (18, 28, 30, 31, 34, 45, 58, 66, 83-93), were tossed out and considered 'statistically irrelevant'.[28]

As previously mentioned, the CDC from the outset made it very clear, even on their website, that this two-tier system was for 'statistical purposes only' and not to be the final determinate as to whether or not an individual had Lyme disease. That was to be based on history, tick exposure, clinical symptoms, lab results and physical examinations.[29]

Unfortunately, however, ever since the disease has been deemed reportable by the CDC, physicians have failed to adhere to the actual purpose of the two-tier system and have been using the test to 'diagnose' Lyme disease. We see this in Alex Peterson's case, when his pediatrician used the system to give Alex a 'Not Lyme Disease' diagnosis. Negative Lyme tests, based on the CDC reportable criteria, are interpreted just as Alex's was. According to the CDC, they mean 'not Lyme disease' (NLD). NLD diagnoses are made thousands of times a day throughout the USA by well-meaning physicians, based on a flawed understanding of the test's actual purpose. Patients with clinical symptoms that 'scream' Lyme disease are misdiagnosed with NLD when the testing comes back negative. The bewildered patient is sent away with no treatment, or a short, ineffectual course of antibiotics.

A closer look at the testing systems

As if this were not bad enough, the two-tier system that depends completely on antibody production is inherently flawed. Why? Because there are far too many ways in which antibody production by the immune system can be evaded by the brilliant *Borrelia burgdorferi*. Some of these ways include the following.[30] The spirochete can:

1. enter tissue cells, including white blood cells, and therefore be protected from antibody immune detection.
2. produce and shift to 'biofilm colonies', clusters of bacteria surrounded by an immunologically impermeable matrix. These bacteria can change their status to 'persisters' and are protected from immune system detection.
3. alter the proteins on its outer surface coat and avoid immune system detection.
4. metamorphose completely and change into what is known as a 'cystic' form. This protective cyst is immune-impenetrable and remains dormant in the patient's system for long periods of time. These cystic forms are capable of regenerating a new generation of spiral motile spirochetes.
5. metamorphose into cell-wall-deficient forms, thus evading immune detection.

Evidence-based medicine and the danger of the logical fallacy

The following represents the prevailing medical opinion as it relates to Lyme disease:

Prevailing medical opinion:

- *All positive IgM antibody tests equal presence of the designated bacteria.*
- *A positive Western Blot antibody IgM test designates an active Lyme infection with clinical symptoms prevailing.*
- *A negative Western Blot antibody test therefore designates no Lyme infection, in spite of clinical symptoms prevailing.*

Of course, given what we know about how *Borrelia burgdorferi* can hide, this is a misleading statement, and absolutely not true. At the same time, it is an excellent example of a 'logical fallacy'. The premises here are 'incorrect', and therefore they lead to a false conclusion. A negative Western Blot Lyme test does not rule out the diagnosis of Lyme disease. Above all else, Lyme is absolutely, and without equivocation, a clinical diagnosis. Yet throughout the medical world, this 'logical fallacy' has led to untold numbers of misdiagnosed and untreated patients.

This is a form of 'deductive' reasoning. There is, however, an alternative form of reasoning – namely, 'inductive reasoning' or 'case-specific reasoning'. This starts with the individual patient's history, symptoms and signs and works from this 'information set' to create a diagnosis. This method of thinking 'inductively' considers the 'particularity' of the individual, which of course involves greater probability and uncertainty. In this case, the truth of the premises does not guarantee the truth of the conclusion. If clinicians confuse the fundamental difference between deductive and inductive reasoning, the resultant error is an over-reliance on evidence-based medicine and the danger of incorporating the 'logical fallacy' trap and reaching false conclusions. The primary reason for this is that the average doctor is working under far too many false assumptions. Below is a list of some of these false premises doctors may be operating under when looking at a case like Alex Peterson's:

1. *Borrelia burgdorferi* is a spiral-shaped spirochetal bacterium that causes Lyme disease; its form remains fixed and does not convert into other structures.
2. Cystic forms and cell-wall-deficient (CWD) forms of *Borrelia burgdorferi* are often found in microscopic examination, mixed together with spirochete forms. In these cases, the cystic forms and CWD forms are considered to be debris only, and not alternative structural forms of the spirochete bacteria.
3. A positive lgM Western Blot test indicates active infection with Lyme disease. A positive test that is reportable to the CDC has antibody production to two out of three of the following identified bands 23-25, 39, 41. Otherwise it is considered a negative test, and therefore assumed that the patient is not infected with Lyme disease.
4. A negative test lgM that has fewer than two positive bands 23-25, 39 and 41, should not be reported to the CDC as it is assumed that the patient is not infected.
5. A patient with fewer than two reportable bands 23-25, 39 and 41 does not have Lyme disease.
6. A symptomatic patient with a positive Lyme test should be automatically treated for no more than three weeks with doxycycline.
7. A symptomatic patient with Lyme-like symptoms but a negative Lyme test should not be treated with three weeks of doxycycline.
8. A positive Lyme test determines whether or not a symptomatic patient has Lyme and needs to be treated.

There is now a third way of medical reasoning. There exists a blend of deductive and inductive reasoning which is termed 'abductive' reasoning, a term coined by the philosopher Charles Pierce. This method of problem solving is used frequently in clinical medicine. It can be understood as applying the hypothesis that best suits and explains the available evidence. When I encounter for the first time a patient I suspect of having Lyme disease, I do not go forward rigidly following the orthodox guidelines.

Lyme and controversy

With families like Alex's (or perhaps like your own), when you start to consider the possibility of a Lyme diagnosis, understand that the diagnosis and treatment of tick-borne disease are extremely controversial in conventional medical circles. After almost 35 years, physicians in endemic areas do not yet have accurate methods to make an exclusive laboratory diagnosis of Lyme disease. After analyzing thousands of serum specimens over 30 years, I have found the laboratory results for Borrelia and other tick-borne infective organisms, as tested by the large laboratories (Quest, Smith Kline, LabCorp), to be inconsistent with the positive clinical evidence of borreliosis. These labs, possibly because of their volume, cannot be relied upon to provide serological confirmation in most cases.

Inter-lab reliability can also be frustratingly inconsistent. I regularly send out blood samples taken from the same patient at the same time to different labs and receive different results from each.

Having reached out to managing directors from three Quest and two LabCorp locations around New York City, we have yet to receive comment on these inconsistent test results.

Other smaller, specialty laboratories tend to be, on the other hand, more accurate and more consistent in their results. They deal almost exclusively with virology, bacteriology and tick-borne infections. Some of these labs include Igenex, Armin Labs,

Stonybrook, iSpot, Medical Diagnostic Lab and Immunosciences. As a patient, you are able to order tests from many of these labs on your own, and can simply bring the kit to your physician/family practitioner, or to anywhere that will do a blood draw in order to run the test.

On average, it takes patients seeing five to 10 different doctors from multiple specialties to obtain a proper diagnosis. Labs like the ones listed above, or like the new test from Armin Labs, TickPlex, are working to counter those numbers. TickPlex, available to patients around the world on request (see Chapter 19 by Dr Armin Schwartzbach later in this book), is the only test currently that looks for Borrelia as well as other microbial agents (Babesia, Bartonella, Mycoplasma, Ehrlichia, etc) in one blood test. This test reports 95 per cent sensitivity and 98 per cent specificity. TickPlex is an exciting new option and is only one of the many new technologies being developed to help improve diagnosis of tick-borne disease.

Follow-up methods for testing treatment 'in progress' would also be of inestimable value, but, at this time, they are not yet commercially available. This leaves the physician in a quandary. Without the serological confirmation of patient improvement, only the physician's clinical judgment, and the patient's regular reporting of symptoms (improving or worsening), can determine treatment outcome. Close monitoring (i.e. the patient keeping a journal), and follow-up visits spaced no more than a month to a month and a half apart, are in reality the only information that the physician has to go on to render a judgment about the progress of treatment.

Things to look out for would include:

- the appearance of co-infection symptoms
- Jarisch-Herxheimer reactions (toxic release from killed bacteria causing exacerbation of symptoms)
- sensitivity to medications
- dosage changes

antibiotic changes
route of administration changes
being referred to specialists for second opinion
(neurology, cardiology, etc).

Even given the updates in the new ICD-11 from the World Health Organization, as they now stand the clinical and laboratory guidelines for the diagnosis of Lyme disease are dangerously misleading.

Other helpful studies, other than antibody assays, have been used to aid the diagnosis of Lyme disease. Sophisticated neuropsychological evaluation can reveal areas of basic brain function and integration, which may be surprisingly abnormal. Frequently, one finds auditory processing deficits, short-term memory deficits, decreased processing speed, concentration and attention deficient issues, and diminished IQ (as compared with previous test scores) in cognitively challenged individuals.

The MRI, and in particular the SPECT scan, are both neuroradiologic diagnostic tools which can show underlying organic brain pathology. Damaged brain tissue demonstrated by the MRI and visualized on a SPECT scan may help delineate the possible extent of the neuropathology. In some instances of Lyme encephalopathy, where diseases like multiple sclerosis (MS) or ALS (amyotrophic lateral sclerosis, another progressive neurodegenerative disease) are considered, a lumbar puncture and examination of the cerebrospinal fluid (CSF) can be helpful in delineating difficult cases.

In cases like Alex's, when you are working with a doctor whom you trust, this can be a real dilemma. There is an intense pressure for families to trust their own physicians. They have made the right judgment call over and over again, but now believe that the presentation of symptoms is not related to tick-borne disease.

The American Academy of Pediatrics, the Infectious Disease Society of America, and more, have all stated very clearly where they stand on the issue of Lyme and tick-borne disease. Even if you, or your child, are displaying symptoms that would be considered red flags for an LLMD (Lyme-literate doctor), your physician is likely to walk away from this diagnosis, moving forward on a 'wait and see' course of treatment that they believe is best for the patient.

If your trusted family physician or specialist has considered Lyme and the testing has been negative, can we ask them to consider a tick-borne diagnosis, in spite of what they believe to be evidence against this possibility? Is there a way to approach this problem differently?

In time, it is my hope that these inaccuracies and inconsistencies in the diagnosis of Lyme and other TBDs will become a thing of the past. Early diagnosis and treatment can transform the lives of those infected.

Chapter 6

Eliza Bedford, age 41
The Lyme maze

Eliza Bedford walked her dog down 3rd Avenue from 86th Street to 79th Street every night at 10 o'clock. It wasn't a long walk, but she loved looking into the shops, dropping into the Whole Foods Market, or sipping a glass of Pino Noir at a local bar along her way. She treasured these contemplative, unhurried timeouts because her life always seemed to be on fast forward.

She worked as a senior physical therapist at NYU Langone Hospital in their rehabilitation department. Every day she was provided with a constant reminder by her physically disabled patients of how appreciative she was of her evening walks, and of how much unrestricted mobility meant to her.

Eliza loved her job. She felt relevant and made a difference to people's lives. She helped them from a condition of severe disability to actual improved functioning. She was particularly moved by several of her patients. There was six-year-old Julie, who had a severe case of cerebral palsy, which had affected her whole body as well as her speech. She was weighed down with heavy braces on her legs and spine so that she wouldn't twist up in grotesque spasms when she attempted to stand up. Eliza worked with her three times a week to help her with equilibrium and balance. Progress was painstakingly slow and laborious, but Julie's cheerfulness and endearing personality made the work feel easy. A 26-year-old war veteran named Riley had served in Afghanistan and lost both his legs in an explosion.

He also displayed remarkable grit and courage in the face of his devastating physical handicap. Eliza worked with him one hour a day, almost every day, to help him accommodate to his new prosthetic legs. That's why she felt so scared when she realized that maybe she was losing control of her own limbs.

It had all started the previous summer, when Eliza took a weekend hiking trip with a few friends up into the Catskills (mountains in southeastern New York). She packed Rusty, her golden retriever, her outdoor camping clothes, her tent and gear into her car and drove out of the city. The weekend was predicted to be perfect for camping, weather clear, no rain. Late August was one of her favorite times of the year. Normally, she'd come home from such a trip totally refreshed and exhilarated. However, after this particular excursion, something felt off. Nothing she could put her finger on exactly – she just felt a little more fatigued and achy than usual.

By late September, Eliza started having consistent muscle soreness and more fatigue. She didn't have the energy to chase her dog Rusty up the stairs to her third floor walk-up. Eliza was exhausted, almost too tired to go on her evening walk. In addition, she was experiencing sharp pain in both knees and hips. 'That's strange,' she thought. 'I don't remember hurting them at any point. I'm overextending myself at work,' she thought to herself. 'That's probably why it hurts. Too much lifting and bending.' She'd stop walking to give herself a rest and to catch her breath, but the pain persisted. Then, seemingly out of nowhere, she experienced a sudden, searing pain in her right elbow that lasted for three days. As quickly as it had appeared, it disappeared.

It was early November, two weeks before Thanksgiving, when she first noticed the pins and needles in her feet when she took off her shoes after work. During the day, she'd be okay, but by the end of her shift her feet were almost numb. She started soaking them in an activated footbath after work, which helped a little but didn't make the numb sensation disappear. They would still be numb the following morning, and all through the workday there would be periods of return of sensation and then returned numbness. She had no idea when the symptoms would occur or disappear.

One day, after a particularly difficult session with a patient, she dropped a glass of water all over the floor. It was a sudden loss of motor control without advance warning. Her hands simply released the cup. There was no apparent neurological reason. 'I must be rubbing off on you,' Riley joked. 'You're getting as clumsy and elephant-footed as I am. Welcome to the club!'

In spite of her symptoms, Eliza kept working. She never missed a single day at the rehab center, even with her fatigue and generalized pain.

Then, one week after Thanksgiving, she started to experience the disquieting symptom of double vision. It occurred when she tried to read a patient's chart and the words appeared blurred and double. Several days later, the double vision was followed by persistent burning and tingling in her upper arms, both left and right side. Her fatigue persisted. There hadn't been one day in the previous two months when she'd experienced restorative sleep when she awoke in the morning. No matter how early she'd gone to bed the night before, it made no difference to her energy. Even if she slept the whole weekend, hardly moving from her bed, it seemed to make little or no difference. And even worse, she was too exhausted at night to walk the dog. She had no choice but to hire a dog walker. It was a type of exhaustion so profound that she barely had enough energy to think. 'It feels like I'm dying,' she remarked to a colleague late one afternoon. 'Whatever it is, it isn't going away.'

Eliza finally capitulated and, after discussing the problem with her mother, promised to visit a neurologist. She set up an appointment with a highly respected specialist in the NYU hospital network. She was examined thoroughly. Blood tests were drawn for viral illness, rheumatoid arthritis, autoimmune illness, immune deficiency and bacterial infections, including a Lyme test. All were found to be within normal limits. Nothing unusual was determined to explain her symptoms. However, on specific neurological testing by EMG, she was found to have peripheral neuropathy. A skin biopsy revealed 'small fiber demyelinating peripheral neuropathy'. Her MRI showed lesions on her brain consistent with multiple sclerosis (MS). She even agreed to a diagnostic lumbar puncture. The results showed equivocal white cell elevation indicative of possible brain inflammation.

A presumptive diagnosis of MS was made after her symptoms and test results had been analyzed. Her treatment consisted of a short course of Sol Medrol, a steroid, IV and interferon injections. She was also prescribed IVIG (gamma globulin) for a period of six months. The neurologist stated kindly, but emphatically, that the treatment would not cure her illness but would likely slow its progression. MS tended go through periods of activity and remission, sometimes becoming activated under stress. If the symptoms progressed they would consider more Sol Medrol IV infusions. The specialist informed Eliza that she could work at the rehab center just as long as she was strong enough and capable enough to handle her responsibilities with patients, but he cautioned her about tiring herself out. He wanted her to get as much rest as possible.

Unfortunately, her condition did not resolve with treatment, though it did seem to improve for a short while, especially some of her fatigue. She slept better and was not as exhausted in the morning. She felt optimistic, but then it worsened. She began to notice a little slurred speech after a tiring, physically challenging session with a patient. She also had some trouble swallowing. Food began to get lodged in her throat without warning. She had two episodes in May of choking that happened in a two-week period.

To make matters worse, her beloved Rusty woke one morning unable to move his hind legs. She frantically carried her 65-pound dog down the four flights of stairs of her walk-up. She bundled him in an Uber taxi and drove straight to her vet, Dr Kirtz. After examining the animal, he explained to a distraught

Eliza that he was going to keep the dog for several days. He'd seen this condition before and he was sure Rusty would improve completely. He just needed a little time to recover.

'But what's the matter with him? Why can't he stand up?'

Dr Kirtz appeared thoughtful, then asked, 'Do you take your dog out of the city into the country?'

'We love to camp. The Poconos are our favorite spot,' she whispered.

'That's what I thought,' he answered. 'I think your dog has been bitten by a deer tick and is suffering from an infection. We'll see what the blood tests show. We have a test here in the clinic. I'll know in one hour. Just relax.'

The diagnosis came back showing ehrlichiosis (an infection caused by the Ehrlichia bacterium) and Rusty was given an intravenous injection of the antibiotic doxycycline and started on doxycycline tablets.

'Go home,' the vet said, 'get some sleep and come back in 24 hours.'

When Eliza returned after a restless, worried night, she couldn't believe what she saw. Her dog was standing in his cage, wagging his tail furiously.

Psychologically, this incident severely damaged Eliza's self-confidence. As a result of these occurrences she took a six-month leave of absence from work. It hurt her deeply. It was the last thing she had ever thought she would do, but she made her decision on the basis of her tenuous health. She gave up her apartment, sold all her furniture, packed up her belongings and moved back home with her mother in Indiana.

She continued to experience numbness in all her extremities, intermittent slurred speech and infrequent episodes of difficulty swallowing. What was even worse, her joints ached painfully but different joints were affected at different times. Sometimes it was the large joints – her hips, knees, and shoulders – and sometimes the small joints – just her fingers and wrists. The rheumatologist said it was autoimmune arthritis, often associated with MS, and if her pain continued he would prescribe a biological immune inhibitor.

On her return visit to the neurologist, he determined that her symptoms were stable but would continue to exhibit periods of remission and relapse. That was the nature of MS. It could wax and wane like this for years, before possibly getting more intense. There was no definitive cause or cure and only theories as to its etiology (cause). Eliza had to be patient and go with where the symptoms led her. He was certain that with the present rate of research and published papers, as well as new medication trials in 2017, that there would be a significant advancement in the field of neurology that would soon help her.

Without work to shape her daily routine, Eliza focused on restoring her health to the best of her ability. She'd spend afternoons scouring the internet for tips. She especially focused on her food intake and only ate organic, vegetarian and gluten-free in order to improve her symptoms. She was willing to give everything a chance, but her symptoms continued to wax and wane. She felt despondent and hopeless and resigned to being disabled.

The following winter she experienced a serious Strep throat that turned into a nasty bronchitis with a hacking cough that didn't stop. She took a trip to the emergency room and received a short course of antibiotics and was told to hydrate and stay in bed for at least two days. She returned home to follow instructions. Strangely, during the course of her antibiotics, after about five days, exactly the time within which she had finished all six tablets of her treatment, her neuropathy noticeably improved. Based on all of the research she had been doing since leaving work, she didn't understand how her neurological symptoms could improve based on only five days of antibiotic treatment. 'Correlation', she remembered from her statistics class years before, does not necessarily equal 'causation', but still, such a dramatic response in such a short time got her thinking. In addition, her positive change in symptoms lasted for more than a month; then unfortunately they returned to their previous disabling level.

Her internet searches started to shift. She began looking for similar cases of similar changes after antibiotic treatment. On one of these research quests, she came across a paper that drew a connection between MS and Lyme disease, and then another and another, even showing cases where the MRIs were indistinguishable one from another. It was impossible to tell the difference between sclerotic lesions designated as MS and those that were diagnosed as tick-borne disease (TBD). They both looked identical!

Could MS have been Lyme disease misdiagnosed? she wondered. How could her doctors have missed this connection, or not brought it to her attention?

Though the diagnosis for MS had once felt so certain, Eliza now felt she needed to find a second opinion.

Physician analysis: The Lyme maze

The patient that I based this story on ultimately did seek a second opinion, and then a third and a fourth, before finding her way to a Lyme-literate doctor (LLMD) who often refers patients to me. Because Eliza's symptoms did not stabilize with well-known multiple sclerosis (MS) treatments, and because they so mysteriously vanished after a course of antibiotics, this physician questioned whether her 'T1 and T2 intensities with sclerotic lesions' could have been connected to something other than MS. After conducting specialty lab testing, the patient was diagnosed with Lyme and the red-cell parasite, Babesia. She was treated with 10 months of oral, intra-muscular and intravenous antibiotics. Gradually, over time, her symptoms improved, not completely, but enough to go back to work in her hometown – Gary, Indiana.

The antibiotic treatment, in this case, was a flag to the LLMD to look for something new, but a case like this one also sees a number of the 'repeated commonalities' explored in the first section of this book. Physicians could have looked for:

- The camping hobby and her dog Rusty in Upstate New York
- The MRI with sclerotic lesions
- The rapid response to antibiotics of her neurological symptoms
- Her shortness of breath and exhaustion as early symptoms
- Her atypical joint pain, with her neurological symptoms
- Her dog's sudden mysterious illness and response to treatment.

Knowing that we see these types of recurring themes, why is it that so many patients who have cycled through doctor after doctor find themselves stumbling onto a Lyme diagnosis?

I see the medical world, especially as it relates to tick-borne disease, as a kind of maze. Patients know they are lost, and are determined to find their way back to health, but every turn leads them down a path that may be taking them in the wrong direction. Think about Eliza's visits to each specialist she saw. What did that visit entail? A visit to a doctor or hospital, testing (that likely came back negative or inconclusive), and a referral to a new doctor that might be able to better understand her situation. The cycle repeated itself over and over again, sending Eliza down different paths without a clear vision of where she was going to end up.

Patients in situations like Eliza's are reminiscent of disoriented train travelers in a Kafka-like scenario. The traveler wishes to board a train on the East Coast with the intention of reaching the West Coast. However, once arrived at the train station, s/he can't find the 'right boarding track' (platform). The information given to him/her concerning 'schedules and time' is hopelessly 'outdated' and inaccurate. In addition, the information booth official continues to direct him/her to the wrong gate. The conductor on the platform denies the existence of such a train ever traveling to the West Coast. The traveler, hopelessly confused, finally boards the correct train that appears to head to the West Coast. Halfway through the journey, s/he is told that his/her destination has been reached. S/he is instructed to get off the train. Little wonder, the 'traveler'/patient is disoriented, feels crazy and begins to doubt the reality of his/her own senses. After all, if the supposed successful course of treatment does not work, the patient's symptoms are no better off at the end than they were at the beginning.

This phenomenon – what I call getting lost in the Lyme maze – regularly consumes patients around the world, especially in locations where Lyme is not considered in the early phase of diagnosis (see Chapter 20 by Dr McManus on the state of Lyme disease in Australia). And what's more troubling is that, even after patients have found themselves out of the the labryith with the correct diagnosis, the debate still rages around proper treatment and leaves patients lost in yet another, new maze – that of the Lyme world itself.

The great Canadian physician Sir William Osler, was the father of bedside, clinical teaching at Johns Hopkins in the early 1900s. He stated:

> *Let not your conception of misfortunes of disease come from work heard. Learn to see, learn to hear, learn to feel. And then know by practice alone can you become experts.*

There needs to be a serious and non-prejudicial re-evaluation of this enigmatic disease state. In the US, the changes must begin with the National Institutes of Health (NIH) and Centers for Disease Control and Prevention (CDC) at the highest level of governmental responsibility. This same information must be communicated to the Department of Health at the state level and to all major insurance carriers, especially in the Northeast, Midwest and California in the US, and in countries around the world. Both the diagnosis and the treatment of what 'informed practitioners' (LLMDs) around the country and the world have designated as 'chronic' or 'persistent' Lyme disease (with or without co-infection) needs to be recognized rather than dismissed out of hand. Perhaps this will be our first step in helping people to find their way out of the Lyme maze.

Chapter 7

Sarah Trindell, age 68
Patient dismissal

Sarah stood on the deck of her backyard sunporch on Staten Island, NY, and surveyed her flower garden. 'This is my quiet little piece of heaven right here,' she thought. 'I wouldn't trade it for any other place I know.'

As a retired schoolteacher, seven years a widow, and with two grown children half-way across the country, Sarah had oceans of time with which to indulge herself. She thought she would hate the time alone – as a fifth grade teacher she had been very active in so many young lives for so long. In her 30-year career she had spent literally thousands of hours in the classroom, at home doing lesson plans, and on the grassy playing field as a coach of the junior varsity soccer team. Still, she didn't mind the time by herself. She would smile through the afternoons as she brushed the coat of her 11-year-old half-collie rescue dog, Brenda-Lee, a constant companion since her husband had died suddenly after a heart attack seven years before.

All through the three seasons, and into the winter when possible, Sarah worked in her half-acre plot, digging, weeding, pruning, planting, seeding, picking and mulching, everything having to do with her garden. She was particularly proud of her herbs and vegetables.

One evening, while deeply engrossed in one of her favorite quiz shows, she felt something vaguely itchy on her upper right thigh. She scratched it a bit, and then left it alone, hardly thinking about it. The next day in the shower, she noticed a red, raised rash spreading out about 3-4 inches or so from the center.

'Doesn't look like any kind of bullseye rash to me,' she thought to herself. She had had at least two of them in the past 10 years, so figured she would recognize another. Sarah had been bitten twice. Twice that she knew with certainty. On one occasion her 'tell-tale sign' had been the infamous 'bullseye rash' on her thigh, and once she had found a tiny, attached 'nymph tick' no bigger than the head of a pin under her breast.

On several occasions over the years she had found female adult ticks crawling in her bed, and she had pulled dozens from her dog over the years. Unfortunately, the yard seemed to attract them. She had tried to be extra careful and always used insect repellant on herself when she worked in the garden. Brenda-Lee always wore a natural bug-repellant dog-collar.

During her past two episodes, several years apart, Sarah had taken herself to the emergency room. The emergency room doctor at the Staten Island hospital had treated her immediately both times. He seemed to know exactly what he was doing. He checked the area thoroughly and had carefully removed the tick with special tweezers.

'Should I have some blood tests. Or test the tick? How would I know if I've been infected?' she had asked with obvious concern.

'Too early for blood tests; won't show a darn thing. Antibodies have to form and that takes at least three weeks.' The doctor had spoken authoritatively. 'As far as sending the tick for testing, the whole issue is academic as far as I'm concerned,' he had said, 'because I'm going to treat you anyway, no matter what the results. Two weeks of doxycycline and you'll be good as new'. Sarah had felt relieved. She had taken the two weeks of the antibiotic and done very well. She had experienced almost no symptoms, just a little intestinal upset when she was taking the medication. Then she had forgotten all about the incident and gone about her business in good health for four years.

The rash this time, she felt sure, was not a bullseye rash. It was light red, had no distinct boundaries and no shape. 'More like a birthmark,' she thought. 'Certainly not like the bullseye I had before.'

A few days later, the rash had disappeared, but Sarah began having strange symptoms. While bending or standing up in her garden, especially if it was too quickly, she would suddenly feel light-headed, dizzy and off balance. Her heart would start to speed up, and she felt as if she might black out. The palpitations were associated with chest pain and shortness of breath. A couple of times in fact, she had tried to stand up from a kneeling position and fallen forward, off balance. It was at this same time that she began to suffer from episodes of vertigo and nausea, associated with excruciating pressure headaches. They weren't exactly migraines, but the pressure build-up was so strong that she felt her head was trapped in a vice. She tried an over the counter migraine medicine, but it didn't help her much and she was determined not to take stronger medication.

Another month went by. Instead of her symptoms improving as she had hoped, they actually worsened. New ones also appeared. Her hip joints and knees became very sore, especially the right knee, and although it was not swollen it was very painful to walk any distance without having to stop and rest. In addition, she began to have difficulty walking up the stairs to her bedroom. She had to stop at least twice to mount her 20 stairs. She had difficulty breathing, and actually had to sit down on the stairs to catch her breath. Her leg muscles felt like she had run a marathon. Her calves were cramping up and the soles of her feet were all knotted up to the point that she could hardly walk freely from one room to the next.

A week later, when it was time to walk Brenda-Lee, she couldn't find her dog's leash. She always left the leash on the wall peg, and now it was gone. Was her mind playing tricks on her?

She spent more than an hour searching for it, practically turning the house upside down. Finally, she absent-mindedly opened the refrigerator door to get some orange juice and there it was, the missing leash, lying neatly rolled up in a Tupperware bowl.

At that very moment, while the leash was dangling mockingly on her wrist the phone rang. It was her oldest daughter, Kathy.

'So, what do you think?' Sarah heard the soft, soothing voice of her daughter on the other end of the line.

'Think about what?' Sarah asked, irritably.

'About the trip?'

'What trip?' Sarah asked again, her irritation growing steadily. There was silence at the other end of the line for several seconds.

'Mom, the kids, us? Tomorrow we are coming out to stay with you for a week. It's the Easter break, remember? You haven't forgotten about it, have you?'

Sarah had forgotten. Her daughter's visit had flown straight out of her head. She was devastated. Sarah was in Dr Peer's office, her family doctor of 20 years, the very next day. She sat nervously on the exam table, a thousand questions flooding through a blizzard of anxious thoughts.

She thought she was getting Alzheimer 's disease. Either that or she was losing her mind. She broke into tears when Dr Peer came into the examining room. Sarah recounted to him the whole history of all her physical symptoms, and her memory decline over the previous six months. He listened carefully; examined her thoroughly and drew six vials of blood; then recommended an MRI at a future date.

'One thing is for sure,' said the doctor, 'you don't have Alzheimer's disease. You drew the clock face just fine and had only a few little errors on your mental status. There were a couple of vice presidents you didn't remember and you had a few calculation errors in serial sevens, but you were perfectly normal on the proverbs and abstract thinking.'

'So, you mean, I just have to live with it? Getting older is your diagnosis for all of these symptoms?'

'I'm afraid so. Aging happens to all of us,' he said kindly.

'I'm afraid it's a terminal illness. Stop worrying so much.'

But Sarah was not convinced, even though she trusted Dr Peer and most of the time his judgment on her medical conditions had been correct.

'Dr Peer,' she said quietly, 'it's more than the memory thing. All my physical symptoms, they can't all be aging. Maybe the Lyme is back. Everyone knows it can recur. And I had that strange rash with the strange bite... Maybe it was an infected tick bite after all?'

He'd already drawn blood to test for Lyme disease.

A week passed and the test results that came back were negative: a negative ELISA 0.5 and CDC negative Western Blot, but 41 IgM and IgG 41, 58, 83-93. She was convinced that those numbers must mean something. Dr Peer explained that 'because you have band markers does not mean that you have a positive test. It only means that you have been exposed to Lyme bacteria sometime in the past. It's protecting you now. Much like a vaccine.'

Sarah's symptoms continued to escalate. Getting lost on her way to the grocery store, forgetting to turn off the oven after cooking, or leaving the dog outside without remembering to bring her in at night were all becoming almost daily occurrences. Kathy and her other daughters started to worry she wasn't safe living alone at home, and began to look into nursing homes or visiting nurses, but the costs were prohibitively expensive.

As Sarah's memory continued to worsen, her mental health went with it. Lost in a dark sea of depression, she was spending most of the day in bed, refusing to delve into her daily routine out of fear that she would somehow get lost along the way.

When Kathy took her mother back to see Dr Peer again, anxious for a referral to a neurologist, the doctor was shocked by Sarah's rapid decline. For her age, this kind of sudden-onset dementia was extremely uncommon. Kathy asked again about the Lyme test, but again was told that her band markers did not signify a positive test result.

Kathy had kids of her own, and between caring for her mother and getting the kids back and forth from school, she needed to call in some help during the day. A kind home nurse by the name of Cynthia was with her each day from 2:00 to 5:00 pm, so Kathy could pick up her kids and work with them on homework. One afternoon Cynthia pulled Kathy aside to express concern about Sarah's diagnosis – it just didn't look like a dementia case to her. She'd seen so many before, and the pattern of events didn't make sense. Cynthia asked if Kathy had considered a possible Lyme diagnosis and handed her a card with the name of a doctor she had heard speak years before.

'I've seen cases like your mother's before,' she said. 'Call him.'

Sarah had already been treated for Lyme multiple times over. Shouldn't those treatments have sufficed? And if they hadn't – why not?

Physician analysis: Patient dismissal

The medical community, for the most part, has been cautioned to avoid 'over diagnosis', thinking that, as well as dangerous, and costly, over-use of long-term antibiotics carries risks. Peer-reviewed journals (*Journal of the American Medical Association (JAMA), The New England Journal of Medicine, the Lancet* and the *British Medical Journal (BMJ)*) have warned against inappropriate antibiotic therapy.[31] As a result, the persistent, kaleidoscopic tick-borne disease syndrome doesn't make sense to a 'cautious, conservative medical mind', which prides itself on 'scientific objectivity'. Borrelia, especially with co-infection, 'blurs' the boundaries and complicates the initial diagnosis, and subsequent treatment recommendations, for the patient.

This is hyper-relevant when thinking about cases like Sarah's. The identification of chronic or persistent Lyme is very unlikely in today's medical climate, unless the physician is properly educated in identifying this syndrome. Chronic tick-borne disease is invariably excluded from the patient's differential diagnosis, particularly if the serology (blood test) produces negative results. Indeed, the presentation of the 'acute phase' of the illness is really the only utilized definition for Lyme disease proper. This definition in actual practice recognizes, almost exclusively, the dermatological and rheumatological symptoms – that is, the rash and the muscle/joint pain [32]

Another theme that stands out in Sarah's case is the importance of the subjective world of the patient. Though her memory lapses could have been attributed to vascular dementia or Alzheimer's, these are not the only conditions that explain this kind of neurocognitive trouble. Unfortunately, the offerings of the patient's 'mind' are normally dismissed as inconsequential, unless the individual is severely disturbed (with psychosis, panic attacks or bipolar). The subjective description of a 'self' in distress is not accepted as helpful or useful diagnostic information. For that reason, the neurological, neuroendocrine, neuropsychiatric and neurocognitive symptoms of 'chronic, persistent Lyme' are almost always overlooked. They are overlooked because they do not appear to be included in most physicians' diagnostic understanding of this complicated phase of the disease. Ask most doctors what constitutes 'chronic Lyme' – namely, how is it diagnosed and treated – and the answer almost always comes back, 'Chronic Lyme does not exist.'

But Sarah's is the first case we have visited where a previous Lyme diagnosis ultimately shaped her treatment path. In cases like Sarah's, it can take years to find the root cause of suffering because of the consistent mainstream dismissal of the possibility of persistent infection. And this is not where the problems stop.

When patients return to Lyme treatment for the second, or sometimes third and fourth time, they are forced to come up against a new form of denial, this time from the insurance companies, some of the biggest players in this debate to shape the experience of patients around the United States. Later in the book, we will hear in more detail about how this form of denial influences the experiences of patients in countries around the world.

Lyme and the insurance battle

In the US in 2012, the House Foreign Affairs Committee of the Infectious Diseases Society of America (IDSA) stated the following:

> *The IDSA recognizes that Lyme disease can be painful and that the disease is not always properly identified or treated* [and later goes on to say] *We sympathize with these patients' suffering, but remain concerned that a diagnosis of so-called Chronic Lyme Disease, suggesting that active infection is ongoing, is not supported by scientific evidence and, more alarmingly, the treatment of long-term antibiotic therapy will do patients more harm than good.*[33]

They go on to state that a majority of Lyme disease cases are 'successfully treated with 10-28 days of antibiotics', and that 'long-term antibiotics have not been found to effectively treat symptoms that persist after the initial infection has cleared.' Their position has not notably changed since this 2012 statement, now more than seven years old.

Insurance companies in the United States take their cue from the guidelines set forth by the IDSA and CDC, and, as a result, are not required to cover treatment that surpasses the 28 days recommended by the IDSA. Even diagnostics are not always covered by insurance. In Aetna's 2017 summary of health insurance coverage for Lyme, efforts as simple as 'antigen detection', 'Borrelia culture' and '*Borrelia burgdorferi* antibody index testing' are listed as 'experimental and investigational because there is inadequate scientific evidence to prove their usefulness in a clinical practice'.[34]

The biggest danger in this refusal to cover treatment is that it forces most, if not all, Lyme-literate doctors (LLMDs) to leave the hospital and mainstream medical system to start practices of their own, where they do not take insurance and patients are forced to pay out of their own pockets for both their care and their treatment.

These doctors, myself included, do their best to submit insurance claims to providers and ask for as much coverage as possible for their patients. Every company, and even every case, is treated differently by the insurance companies. I know of patients who have had years of treatment covered by insurance, and others who have been cut off after only one round of antibiotics. This lack of consistency only makes things more confusing and troubling for patients, who now must add a new component – of information proficiency and self-advocacy – to their experience of serious infection.

If we return to Sarah's case for a moment, the importance of this type of self-advocacy becomes clear. Without the intervention from her nurse, Sarah's symptoms would have continued to worsen. She would have gotten sicker and sicker, without a clear understanding of what was causing her suffering. Thanks to the intervention of her nurse, Sarah was able to seek out a second opinion. But then again, another problem comes to light. Having already been treated for Lyme disease multiple times before, would this LLMD be able to get insurance coverage for Sarah's treatment? Likely not. The limited thinking on cases such as this prevents patients from receiving the care they need and deserve.

Chapter 8

Matt Ravenhall, age 29
Treatment: the nuts and bolts

Matt Ravenhall graduated '*cum laude*' from Ohio State in business and finance. He was popular with both men and women and he had an engaging personality that could win you over immediately, yet was also unassuming, generous and completely genuine. His future appeared wide open. Matt seemed destined for success.

One month after he graduated with his Master's degree, he was offered a lucrative paying position, as a financial analyst with one of the three top investment firms on Wall Street. For a graduate student, just out of college with zero work experience, the job and salary he was offered were astronomical. He was excited by the offer and accepted immediately without interviewing for any other position. It was the type of position that allowed him to assimilate new practical financial information, something that the business school could never teach him. From the very first day he was swept up in a whirlwind of activity. He quickly made work friends and within two weeks met Melissa, a sweet, Juilliard graduate in piano music working part-time as a waitress. They bonded immediately. He also found a spectacular apartment in Williamsburg, Brooklyn, that the two of them could afford together, and signed a two-year lease. He was even thinking about buying a BMW roadster, which he had coveted for years.

Matt bought the car that very same day and he and Melissa took full advantage of their new-found freedom and mobility.

They drove all over the Northeast, stayed at B&Bs, slept in the car near the shore in the Hamptons, slept out in sleeping bags on the beach in Nantucket, drove and hiked in Maine as well as in the New Hampshire White mountains. It was a glorious summer and fall and Matt felt on top of the world.

Approximately one year passed from his arrival in New York. Matt was doing excellently at work. He and Melissa were living together with almost no adjustment problems and were continuing to spend their weekends taking camping and car trips all over the Northeast. Matt had also received a substantial raise over the past year and was appointed account manager for a teachers' huge pension fund. He was well respected by everyone and his career showed great promise.

It was when Matt was celebrating his 34th birthday with Melissa and six other friends that he suddenly, and without warning, experienced a wave of severe dizziness and nausea. He was afraid to stand up because he felt like he was going to fall over onto the table. Then, as he tried to get up from his chair, he was struck by a severe, blinding headache that almost threw him to the ground. He excused himself, trying to control the need to vomit, and wobbled unsteadily to the men's room, where he threw up his whole birthday dinner.

He returned to his friends' table and apologized for the scene he had created. He excused himself from the group and told them he wasn't feeling terrible.

When he got back to the apartment he threw himself across the bed without taking off a stitch of clothing. He fell into a deep coma-like sleep that lasted more than 18 hours. When he woke up, Melissa was standing over him anxiously. He felt completely 'out of it'. The terrible pressure headache was somewhat better, but it definitely had not gone away. Unfortunately, it continued almost all day, along with the dizziness and light-headedness.

For the first time in a year he took three days off sick from his work and did nothing but sleep and flop around the apartment aimlessly and then sleep hours more. After the second day, several new symptoms popped up. He experienced blurred vision and sound sensitivity, something that had never happened to him before. He complained that the TV was hurting his eyes and the sound of Melissa's hair dryer was almost intolerable. Also, the sound of her electric toothbrush made him feel crazy. And then there was Melissa chewing and cracking gum while she was doing the dishes. This had used to amuse him and they had joked about it often. Now it was so annoying and distracting that he had to leave the room while she was doing it.

After his third sick day, he felt somewhat better and tried to go to work. He arrived late, avoided talking to most of his friends and sat down immediately in front of his computer. He was there for less than an hour, but in that short time Matt became overwhelmed by the barrage of stimuli. Brokers calling out trades, phones ringing off the hook, clients wanting information, irritating music in the background, florescent lights glaring overhead, copy toner smells, harsh perfume... All of it overwhelmed him. He got up from the computer screen, with a thundering headache that felt like his brains were going to blow apart. He threw some documents into his briefcase and, without speaking to anyone in the office, just fled the scene.

Four months went by and Matt was feeling horrible. Everything hurt like crazy: his muscles and joints, the base of his thumb, his rib cage seemed so inflamed that it was hard for him to breathe. One night it was so bad he felt he was having a heart attack. He took himself to a walk-in clinic and they reassured him that he had no heart problems, only costochondritis. The chest pain over the next few weeks seemed to improve, but his neck was so stiff and locked up that turning it was pure agony. Then his lower back seemed to be perpetually in spasm. He needed at least two pillows to sit at his computer desk. And to him the most damaging change of all was the fact that he couldn't remember things from one day to the next. That included what he had done, who he had spoken to, what he had read – sometimes even forgetting what day it was. It seemed as if the flow of events that he experienced day to day was wiped clean every 24 hours

Perhaps it was the stress of his persistent physical symptoms that weren't improving, or having to live up to unreasonable expectations at work, or even his relationship with Melissa seemed to be unraveling day by day. Matt's good nature and sunny disposition appeared to have vanished overnight. One evening, he had raged at Melissa, calling her a 'lazy slob' for not doing the laundry on Saturday. He seemed completely out of control. She was reduced to tearful sobbing. He started to apologize. It was the third time in less than one month that he had blown up and lost it with her. Before he could apologize she ran from the TV room and went into their bedroom. She threw all of her things into two large suitcases and wheeled them out of the apartment.

Matt stared straight ahead, not saying a single word. He remained silent as the door slammed loudly behind her. A shock wave of anxiety swept over him, like nothing he had ever felt before. He broke into a drenching, total body sweat, like the ones he had been having at night over the previous few months. He had commented to Melissa previously that he felt like he was drowning in his own sweat. He had soaked his sheets right through to the mattress.

After Melissa had left he felt saddened but not devastated. He needed to be alone. Living with another human being took work and energy. He hardly had enough stamina to get up every morning and go to work on time. One evening he noticed that climbing up the stairs was becoming sheer torture, almost impossible to get up a flight without puffing for air, holding on to the rail and stopping in the middle to catch his breath for great, heaving gasps and gulps of air.

He reached out to a pulmonologist at Lennox Hill Hospital, who ordered an MRI of Matt's chest.

'Everything looks absolutely clear,' he said. 'No lung lesions, no thickening, no prominent nodes. Everything looks perfect. Don't worry so much. It will pass as mysteriously as it came.'

But Matt wasn't satisfied with the explanation. He went to see a cardiologist, Dr Winston Marian, who did a complete cardiac work-up, including stress testing, ultrasound and an EEG. All the tests came back negative.

'You have a perfectly healthy heart. There is nothing to worry about,' said the physician. 'You finance guys are all the same. Stress, stress and more stress. Just slow down. You'll be fine.'

Matt was pleased that both doctors were thorough and complete. They had taken sufficient time with him, to hear him out. Matt appreciated the thoughtfulness of their approach, but he wasn't satisfied.

'If everything is okay, why am I feeling this way? Why do I have all these symptoms that come and go and then come back and never leave me? This has never happened to me before.'

The doctor thought for a moment and said diplomatically, 'I'm not a psychiatrist, but I think you've been way over-doing it at work and in your personal life. You're still adjusting to the rhythm of the city. And breaking up with your girlfriend doesn't help at all. If I remember my psych seminars, what you have is called GAD – generalized anxiety disorder. An antidepressant may do wonders for you, along with a beta blocker for the palpitations and what we call dysautonomia – deregulation of the nervous system. It can replicate all your symptoms.'

Matt left the office a little unsure. He didn't completely understand everything the doctor had said to him, but he was happy to get some closure and an explanation for his persistent symptoms.

He knew what to do: he'd sign up at the gym and begin to work out in earnest. He was definitely out of shape. Maybe he'd call Melissa and tell her what the doctor had said to him. And definitely try to get back together again.

And yes, maybe he'd see a therapist and even try some medication for anxiety. As for his remaining nagging symptoms, well, he would just put them out of his head. He could do that now that he knew what caused them.

'Dys-auto-nomia,' he said out loud. 'Isn't that something?"

After the diagnosis, Matt left his finance job and made focusing on health his full-time job. He worked out as much as he could, started seeing a therapist, regularly took his medication, ate well, slept well – everything he could control, he did. One afternoon during one of his work-outs, he felt a familiar powerful tightness in his chest followed by a searing pain that seemed to emanate out of his whole body. He fell to his knees, almost unable to breathe, and fainted. He woke up in the ambulance on the way to the hospital, having learned that the gym attendant had called 911.

Before he was discharged, the doctors assured him over and over again that he had not had a heart attack. The tingling he felt in his arms, the tremors, the headaches – the doctors acknowledged these symptoms were uncomfortable but assured him again that they were not overly concerning. He was fine. It was a simple bundle branch block, or a delay or blockage along the pathway that electrical impulses travel on to make your heart beat. This was something that meds could easily cure. But the diagnosis nagged at him. He had been doing everything right, he had been taking care of his body as best he possibly could. He was tired of taking medication for some new diagnosis every month, and that feeling in his chest terrified him.

He went home that night and dived into research about bundle branch blocks, finding a number of studies linking these with an infection – Lyme disease.

After ordering his own Igenex test (see page 261), he discovered that he was indeed infected and not just with Lyme. Tired of doctors and appointments and diagnosis after diagnosis, Matt set out to cure himself. He'd read about people who had done so online with supplements and holistic treatments. If health was his full-time job, he was going to get this under control. He tried to bring himself back to his old way of thinking.

Finding new confidence in this diagnosis that finally seemed to make sense, he thought to himself, 'What can't I do alone?'

Physician analysis: Treatment – the nuts and bolts

As we have already seen, the standard care earnestly followed by most of the well-meaning physicians in the community is unproven beyond the acute phase of Lyme infection.[35] The incomplete science upon which the standard treatment plan rests is, in the final analysis, simply 'speculative hypothesis' spun into treatment recommendations. Though acknowledged in the International Lyme and Associated Diseases Society (ILADS) Guidelines, the guidelines set out by the Infectious Diseases Society of America (IDSA) ignore the critical medical problem of 'advanced borreliosis' from which many patients suffer.

As a result, infected patients like Matt often find themselves on a slow, inexorable, slide to 'chronic unwellness', and a significantly diminished quality of life. In many of the severe cases, the patient may have visited a merry-go-round of no less than half a dozen unsuspecting physicians and specialists before finally being diagnosed and properly treated, if at all.

Many patients, like Matt for example, ultimately turn to self-diagnosis and find their way to Lyme and tick-borne disease without the help of a doctor. Like Matt, they often turn their backs on the medical system and decide to pursue treatment on their own. By doing this, many lose access to the treatment options they may need in order to heal fully. The Lyme bacterium is highly complex, and if not treated properly can cause serious problems in the body.

The Lyme bacterium and the body

In some of the earliest Lyme research, Dr Burgdorfer, the researcher after whom the Lyme Borrelia organism is named, showed that the bacterium had the capability to penetrate cell walls.[36] In his studies, he demonstrated that it invaded the tick's gut wall and spread via its hemolymph to its salivary glands. The following is an overview (albeit a technical one) of the way that this infection can penetrate cells in the body, or evade immune detection.

Binds plasminogen[37]

The Borrelia bacterium binds human plasminogen to surface proteins. It is then converted to plasmin to provide the mechanism whereby it can digest the extracellular matrix and penetrate cell walls using the host's own enzymes.

Blood-brain barrier[38]

Brain microvascular endothelial cells (BMECs) are essential to the blood-brain barrier due to their high electric resistance. Borrelia can traverse this barrier by the addition of plasminogen, which is localized to the site of spirochete-endothelial cell interaction, leading to a transient breakdown of the blood-brain barrier and facilitating the invasion of B. burgdorferi *in the central nervous system. It is evident the Borrelia bacterium is resourceful, if not extremely clever. It has the advantage of millions of years of evolutionary practice, and the necessary equipment to penetrate most cell-types.*

Intracellular survival[39]

Once inside, it can survive within the cytoplasm, safe from immune detection. This would explain one of the possible mechanisms by which the organism escapes the immune system of the 'host' and persists during the later stages of the disease.

Inside macrophages[40]

Also, as stated, persistence of B. burgdorferi *has been shown to exist within migrating macrophages, or immune cells. This provides a possible pathogenic mechanism for recurrent borreliosis.*

Changes surface antigens[41]

The organism can also evade immune detection by changing what is known as its 'surface antigens', a complex protein sequence on its outer coat, and even alter the lipoproteins within its cytoplasm, giving it a survival advantage.

Cystic form[42]

Electron microscopy has revealed that B. burgdorferi *appears to metamorphose from an active, motile, spiral, flagellar form to a dormant, resting cystic form, particularly in the CSF. Under special circumstances, it can then reverse itself from the dormant cystic form back to the active motile form, producing a whole new generation of spirochete bacteria, without a re-infection from a tick bite. Present testing methods, under these circumstances, would be unable to detect the presence of the bacterium in the CSF.*

Elegant photo-microscopy demonstrated that the bacterium can penetrate a T or B cell (lymphocyte) and camouflage itself with the cytoplasmic contents, much the same as wearing a raincoat, to escape immune detection.

Untreated borreliosis in most cases, along with possible co-infection, will eventually become a chronic spirochetal infection, following the example of other bacteria of the same genus: syphilis, relapsing fever and leptospirosis. The corkscrew, mature B. burgdorferi *bacterium, besides exhibiting intracellularly, has been shown in a number of studies to change to a cystic cell-wall-deficient phase, or non-motile spherical starvation stress form, seeming to occur when the host environment becomes hostile, i.e. decreased source of fatty acids and lipids. Remarkably in this state, the bacterium can persist and evade immunologic detection.*

Under times of physical or psychological stress for the patient, the bacterium can produce a new generation of spirochetes. They metamorphose from the cell-wall-deficient form back to the mature, spiral form. If the live B. burgdorferi, *as well as its plasmid structure, or its fragments (flagellar protein), persists in the body, it can still continue to induce tissue injury in the patient.*

Inflammation[43]

The Borrelia bacterium promotes inflammation by stimulating endothelial cells (cell walls of capillaries) to cause white cells (leukocytes) to adhere to them and produce a soluble agent, IL-8, that attracts neutrophils, causing persistent inflammation or, more specifically, vasculitis.

Molecular mimicry[44]

'Molecular mimicry' with autoimmune-like pathology, or the production of a neurotoxin, not yet isolated, liberated by the bacteria, have both been suggested as possible pathogenic mechanisms. Chronic, debilitating, neurological deficits may take months, or even years, to develop (a creeping unwellness). This chronic, persistent, infection over time increases the possibility of an autoimmune-type reaction (a classic immune cascade with release of lymphocyte cytokines and interleukin-2/6). The CNS appears to be particularly susceptible to this type of process (encephalopathy). Other illnesses, such as multiple sclerosis or systemic lupus, have on more than one occasion been suspected of being the result of an underlying Borrelia infection. These are only a small sample of the basic biological facts, relating to the pathogenesis of Borrelia. These facts must be taken into consideration, when treatment program guidelines are recommended, most notably for the chronically infected patient. This issue is far too important to be co-opted by a small handful of IDSA academic physicians.

A closer look at treatment

The usual treatment recommendations are, for the most part, extremely limited. Only minimal selections of oral antibiotics are prescribed: penicillin G, tetracycline, doxycycline and amoxicillin. In addition, the duration of treatment is curtailed long before the presenting symptoms have resolved. Frustrating relapses are a common occurrence after what is considered sufficient treatment. Often the harried physician, who believes he has treated the patient appropriately, can offer nothing but incomplete symptom relief for persistent symptoms, with other prescribed medications. Intravenous therapy, when initiated, usually consists of three to six weeks of antibiotics. Insurance carriers have strict rules governing longer-term treatment, and often refuse to cover these essential requests.[45]

Alternative oral medications may well be a more effective option clinically in patients who have failed to improve on the more commonly prescribed regimens. These new antibiotics include Ceftin, Biaxin, Menacyline and Zithromax. Additionally, a number of anti-parasitic medications are not considered in the IDSA guidelines. They can be effective in counteracting the effects of chronic, relapsing borreliosis.[46]

The usual recommended intravenous medications, as set out in the IDSA Treatment guidelines,[47] include only Rocephin, penicillin G and, sometimes, Claforan. Other options (such as intravenous Zithromax, Merrem, IV Doxycycline, and Vancomycin – the US names) are not utilized but, in practice, can be critical in treating the condition. Combinations of oral medications (i.e. the cephalosporin and / or macrolide antibiotic group combined with an anti-parasitic) or antimalarial medication, though not listed in the guidelines, are extremely helpful against the disease.

Obviously, extended intravenous treatment programs, ranging from three to six months and sometimes up to one year, are not considered by most physicians – and yet, it is clear that without these long-term programs, some patients would be seriously compromised, remain untreated and relapse quickly.

Maintenance antibiotic therapy is not discussed in the guidelines, a vitally important part of any treatment program after intravenous treatment. Almost all extended treatment methods are continually referred to as 'unproven or not medically necessary' by most of the larger insurance companies, aided in no small measure by the consultant specialists whose writings they quote and who they employ to 'support' their frequent denials for care. I must, however, give the devil his due. In my practice, although denials are commonplace, the majority of patients have been approved for 12-16 weeks of intravenous antibiotic therapy, based on my letter of medical necessity.

The trouble with treatment

But, here's the trouble. The truth about treatment is that it is profoundly and essentially problematic. It revolves around 'too much / too little'. We are either painting with too broad a brush, or not painting anything at all.

The too-little approach features doxycycline 100 mg twice a day for three weeks from the Infectious Diseases Society of America (IDSA). The generally held belief is that this cures all presentations of Lyme disease, ranging from early Lyme to patients with an already established history of a known tick bite and persistent symptoms. Anything after that original antibiotic course is left to the 'post-Lyme syndrome' diagnosis – namely, no infection, just long-term healing.

On the other side stands the International Lyme and Associated Diesease Society (ILADS), where too much is the approach. The standard identification of Lyme disease is as an infectious / inflammatory / immunological paradigm with multiple organisms, including, but not limited to: spirochetes, unhealthy gut bacteria, parasites, and more. In a recent NIH-funded study on tick control method, they state that ticks are spreading 'more different kinds of infectious microbes to people and animals than any other arthropod group… The spiral-shaped bacterium that causes Lyme disease is perhaps the best-known microbe transmitted by ticks; however, ticks also transmit infectious agents that cause human babesiosis, anaplasmosis, tick-borne encephalitis and other diseases.'[48] These organisms work together synergistically or endo-symbiotically to form a complex chronic illness affecting every organ in the body. Therefore, treatment, by the very nature of what is being treated, must include a combined therapeutic strategy utilizing an integrated approach, including combinations of antibiotics, antiparasitics, antivirals and antifungals, for extended periods of time. These specific pharmaceuticals can be supported by other medications to help ease symptoms (as mentioned above), but not to the exclusion of the critical extended antibiotic and antiparasitic protocols. Also of great importance is the use of nutraceutical, herbal and detoxification treatments to support the immune system, and reduce inflammation in the compromised patient.

So, what is the conscientious physician to do? Where is he/she to start? Where does one begin to unravel the Gordian Knot?

The problem with the treatment of tick-borne disease is that there is really no guideline or GPS to direct a physician through the maze of symptoms, or even to recognize the syndrome. Every patient is unique, and treatment must be specifically crafted.

It is as if you and the patient have found yourselves in a dark mysterious forest, and it's your job as a caregiver to guide the patient safely through the dangerous terrain to the other side. As a guide, you generally know a lot about the forest, but nothing about what is in the interior. You have no maps or compass for what lies ahead. You have no idea where the swamps lie or where the dangerous animals hide. You only know where you stand as far as north, south, east and west and from these reference points you have to take responsibility to lead the patient to safety.

This journey through the forest will depend on many variables, and all will affect the outcome. For example, the determination of the patient, the experience of the guide, and the bond of trust between the two individuals.

Dr Richard Horowitz released a book titled, *Why Can't I Get Better? Solving the Mystery of Lyme and Chronic Disease*, in 2013. This book has become the guidebook on which many LLMDs base their treatment protocols. In his Appendix A,[49] he lays out protocols for the proper treatment of Borrelia and co-infections. Upon reviewing his recommendations, I found myself more or less in accord with him. I had used almost the same combinations of medications and treatments over my career of treating tick-borne disease. But here is what is remarkable about that fact. I had not read his book until late in 2017. How did I come to the same conclusions about the efficacy of treatment combinations?

In both of our journeys, probably the most influential resource was Dr Joseph Burrascano's guidelines, which he updated and posted freely on the internet beginning in 1985.[50] Or perhaps the Lyme Disease Foundation conferences under the leadership of Karen Forschner, including those of Dr Kenneth Liegner. Other important contributions to treatment over the years were the yearly studies by Sam Danta on the use of long-term medications for the treatment of persistent Lyme, or the thousands of studies published over the past few years and presented at the annual ILADS conference.[51] These have all influenced the way that treatment is conducted.

Yet, with all of this information, the patient and physician still stand at the edge of the forest, preparing to treat what can seem to be a very simple Lyme case. Even without connections or other complications, it can be difficult to know where to start. What dosage of antibiotics should be used, and for how long? By experience, most physicians do not prescribe enough antibiotics and stop far short of eradicating the bacteria. More than 20-30 per cent of patients initially treated with the traditional course of antibiotics (doxycycline) will relapse because the medication is bacteriostatic and will need immune system activity to kill the bacteria.[52]

There is this rigid, almost religious-like belief, in the efficacy of doxycycline for three weeks for any and all presentations of tick-borne disease. In my mind, this is an antiquated and harmful reduction that flies in the face of good science. Instead, a more modern approach to treatment protocols is the use of multiple combinations of antibiotics and anti-parasitics at the same time.

But how does the responsible physician choose which of these combinations work best for their particular patient? Where are the peer reviewed, double-blind matched studies for each combination as compared to a different population?

The answer is nowhere. Nowhere in the literature can you find any reference to the above protocols used by ILADS physicians. By the principles of evidence-based medicine, they don't exist. The current treatment of tick-borne disease syndrome is almost all anecdotal or based on reports of successfully treated Lyme patients by the Lyme treating community.

There is so much published basic science on the pathophysiology of the organisms that make up the Multi Systemic Infectious Disease Syndrome (Horowitz).[53] There is much written about testing, and what a positive or negative test may mean, about how many bands are necessary to correctly diagnose an active Lyme case. The Borrelia genome has been unraveled. The immune system's activity has been declassified. The relationship between the organ system and invasion has been clearly outlined. Yet when it comes to treatment protocols it's the Wild West.

In an article in the *New England Journal of Medicine* entitled 'Tolerating Uncertainty—The Next Medical Revolution?' Simpkin and Schwartzstein wrote the following:

> *We believe that a shift toward the acknowledgement and acceptance of uncertainty is essential for us as physicians, for our patients, and for our health care system as a whole.*
>
> *In medicine today, uncertainty is generally suppressed and ignored consciously and unconsciously. Being uncertain instills a sense of vulnerability in us as physicians. It is unsettling and makes us crave black and white zones to escape this gray-zone space. Our protocols and checklists emphasize the black-and-white of medicine. Doctors often fear that by expressing uncertainty, they will project ignorance to patients and colleagues. So, they internalize it and mask it.*
>
> *By attempting to achieve a sense of certainty too soon, we risk*

premature closure in our decision-making process, thereby allowing our hidden assumptions and unconscious biases to have too much influence and increase the potential for diagnostic error.

As we move further into the 21st century, it seems clear that technology will perform the routine tasks of medicine. Our value as physicians will lie in the gray zone space, where we will have to support patients who are living with 'uncertainty' – work that is essential to strong and meaningful doctor-patient relationships. It is the nature of medicine to be uncertain. And that is alright. We should remind ourselves of Osler's maxim: 'medicine is a science of uncertainty and an art of probability'. Ironically only 'uncertainty' is a sure thing. Certainty is an illusion!

Probably, there is no better example of uncertainty in medicine than the diagnosis and treatment of TBD. From the very definition of what constitutes TBD, to its diagnosis with uncertain testing, to its broad clinical presentation, to its unpredictable and uncertain treatment responses, to the multiple medication options needed to treat the syndrome, to the individualized patient responses, all of these factors over and over, place the doctor-patient relationship squarely in the middle of gray-zone uncertainty!

As already mentioned, the treatment of TBD is much more than just antibiotic or antiparasitic use alone. Medication for insomnia, medication or nutraceuticals for pain relief, for neuropsychiatric difficulties (depression, anxiety), neurocognitive difficulties (ADD, ADHD), endocrine problems (thyroid, adrenal), arthritis, muscular spasms with trigger points (fibromyalgia), weight problems, yeast overgrowth, dietary restrictions, nutritional supplementation for immune-support (a whole complex field in itself and vital to healing), physical therapy prescription and family support are some of the therapeutic interventions that must be considered while treating a tick-borne disease patient.

Bacterial resistance and antibiotic limitations

In a paper published in 2015 in the *International Journal of Molecular Sciences*, the authors Gang Zhou et al described three specific lines of defense by bacteria against antimicrobial agents. 'Antimicrobial resistance' can be defined as an ability of bacteria to resist antimicrobial agents that they were originally sensitive to. These 'resistance factors' were categorized into three groups.[54]

1. Biofilm

The first was the **formation of biofilm**, which can be done by most bacteria to overcome the action of antimicrobial agents. The multi-factor methods employed by biofilms include (but are not limited to):

restriction of penetration of antimicrobial substances within the biofilm

the use of different metabolic rates within the biofilm

gene regulation, and

formation of persister bacteria, which live in a highly protected phenotypic state, grow at different rates, and differentiate similar to spore formation.

These mechanisms contribute significantly to the reduced susceptibility of biofilms to antibiotic agents (likely due to transcriptional programming). Thus, biofilm restricts the penetration of antimicrobial substances, including antibiotics.

There have been some novel approaches used to control biofilms; for example, combinations of tobramycin and clarithromycin have shown clearance of *P. aeruginosa* (pulmonary biofilm) and D-amino acid can be used to inhibit biofilm.

2. Active removal of antibiotics from within cells

The second line of defense is the **cell wall, cell membrane**

and efflux pumps which actively pump the antibiotics out of cells. Thus, the antibiotic in question cannot remain stable and accumulate at the target site in concentrations sufficient to inhibit bacterial survival.

3. Plasmids and chromosomal changes

The third line of defense is when antibiotics do manage to breach the cell wall, the organisms are able to **manipulate 'target sites'** and give rise to **intracellular 'quenchers'**. Plasmids, a small circular, double-stranded DNA molecule in bacterial cells, can replicate independently and can survive in the presence of antimicrobial agents. Plasmids contain a great number of enzymes that can catalyze antibiotics into non-toxic forms. Resistance to penicillin, caused by plasmids, is one such example. Chromosomal changes are another weapon in the arsenal of bacterial resistance. Transposon (the jumping gene) can move from one location in a chromosome to another in the same or a different chromosome. This alters the genetic constitution of the bacteria. (Can you imagine the mischief that goes on amongst bacteria under cover of a biofilm tent? All that gene swapping to protect themselves from our paltry antibiotics!)

Return to Matt's case

Having now shared all of this information, I return to Matt's case. This recurring theme of turning one's back on the medical system after a frustrating search for diagnosis is concerning, especially as we know how much treatment is often needed for a full patient recovery.

The treatment of this disease should also be much more comprehensive than just antibiotic use alone. Issues of sleep deficit medication for insomnia, pain relief for central and peripheral nervous system, neuropsychiatric difficulties (depression, anxiety), neurocognitive difficulties, endocrine problems (thyroid, adrenal), arthritis, muscular spasms with trigger points (fibromyalgia), weight problems, yeast overgrowth, dietary restrictions, nutritional supplementation for immune-support (a whole complex field in itself and vital to healing), physical therapy prescription, family support are some of the therapeutic interventions that must be considered while treating a tick-borne disease patient, all of which would be hard to tackle on your own.

Though I certainly understand this instinct, I would encourage all patients who suspect a potential Lyme diagnosis to reach out for the support of an LLMD or another empathetic physician who will be able to carefully and comprehensively oversee their care.

Chapter 9

Lola Carter, age 21
Identity, the self-system and Lyme patienthood

Lola Carter was the youngest of four sisters, and the first in the family to attend Columbia University on a full scholarship. Her PhD subject was Early American History, and she thoroughly enjoyed the research, writing and small tutorial classes. She'd grown up in a small town in Western Massachusetts, and studying in the Big Apple was a dream come true. She missed her family and the giggles and chatter of her sisters, but she did not miss the almost non-existent town, with its acres and acres of empty fields, one pharmacy and a single grocery store.

Soon after she arrived in New York, she found a part-time job working as a waitress close to the university on the evening shift – six to midnight at a café in Harlem. It was a small hole in the wall, a hangout mostly for Columbia students. It was a friendly kind of place with lots of regulars, many of whom she knew by name and face. She was comfortable joking with them and they all seemed to appreciate her upbeat personality and sense of humor.

At school, her PhD tutorials were intense and demanding, but stimulating. She had no trouble keeping up with the assignments and she was picked to be a teaching assistant for the freshman spring semester. She was regularly complimented on her insights in class and caught the eye of a fellow student, Kevin from New Zealand. They soon developed a chemistry and became romantically involved after three months of almost daily contact. They couldn't get enough of each other. When Lola had time off from the café, they'd take a trip Montauk or Fire Island to explore the outdoors, sometimes even sleeping outside under the stars. Meanwhile, her waitress job was paying enough just with tips alone to splurge on designer jeans and a pair of Italian leather boots down in trendy SoHo.

Her life continued splendidly along the same path for another month or two. Then, one Friday night in March, Kevin and Lola were supposed to meet after her shift at the restaurant, and go to the Village Vanguard to hear a popular Jazz combo. She received a text message from Kevin an hour before he was supposed to pick her up. His father had been taken seriously ill with a stroke that had left him paralyzed. Kevin was leaving the country immediately to care for his dad in New Zealand. He didn't know if and when he was returning to NYC, and as a result, was suspending his PhD studies indefinitely. She tried to call Kevin all through that night, but there was no answer. He had disconnected his phone.

Soon after Kevin's sudden departure everything began to change for her. Slowly at first, almost imperceptibly. At work, she was struggling to keep up with the flow and the fast pace of the café. Her once razor-sharp memory was becoming more and more unreliable. As weeks went by, she became more and more absent-minded and found herself losing focus and constantly daydreaming. She would forget drink orders, and began to mix them up. She brought the wrong food to the wrong table. And though she painstakingly wrote everything down on a pad, she still struggled to remember the orders. And her studies were not going well in her PhD program.

She began missing assignments, falling asleep in her tutorial classes, and just not showing up for her seminars. One Friday afternoon when she had missed her third seminar in a row, her professor called her aside and asked her to come into his office. He told her that he was disappointed in her performance and that she risked losing her scholarship. Was there anything wrong at home that could be distracting her, he asked her kindly. Lola opened up and explained that something strange had happened to her, for sure, something that she had never experienced before.

'I absolutely don't sleep. I have terrible insomnia. But then I can't get out of bed to start my day,' she said. 'I can't seem to wake up.' In addition, she told her professor that her joints and muscles felt like she'd run a marathon. She had pain all over her body, especially her hips and knees. The pain never seemed to go away. It just moved from one place to another, she explained, but the pain remained just as intense. 'And, professor,' she whispered, 'I can't remember a thing. Absolutely nothing.'

Her professor encouraged her to take a trip to the campus health center to get checked, assuring her, 'They're thorough. They'll have a good idea of what's wrong with you.'

After a series of visits, she was diagnosed with Epstein-Barr virus and fibromyalgia. She was prescribed a nerve pain medication and sleeping pills. It helped a little. She slept a bit more and her nerve pain diminished. But over time her exhaustion became more pronounced and her knees were so painful that going up the stairs was an ordeal. Strangely though, they were not swollen.

After a number of specialists, including a rheumatologist, two different neurologists, an internist and a psychiatrist, had all examined her and heard her story, she was pronounced well and fit. 'Probably a severe case of stress,' she was told. Despite this diagnosis, nothing helped her get well. Her symptoms persisted, even worsened.

Nine months after Lola enrolled in her PhD program, she tearfully went to Professor Durst's office, letter in hand, and took a medical leave of absence. She returned home to her small town in Western Massachusetts, exhausted.

When Lola's sisters first saw her, they hardly recognized her. She was gaunt, had lost at least 15-20 lb (6.5-9 kg), and appeared sullen, depressed and beyond exhaustion. She complained daily of intractable migraine headaches, stayed in her room almost constantly with the shades drawn so as to not let in any daylight, and slept more than 12 hours a day, hardly getting up to eat. The bubbly, cheerful, intelligent and optimistic young woman who had left to conquer New York with a scholarship, working towards a PhD from Columbia University was completely debilitated and incapacitated. She looked like she had aged at least 10 years in less than nine months.

It became immediately clear to her family and friends at home that something was seriously wrong. Lola's symptoms continued to worsen. She became more depressed and withdrawn and even at one point was so distraught that she considered suicide. Her pain was constant and the muscle tremors were so intense she was positive that she had ALS (amyotrophic lateral sclerosis or 'motor neurone disease'). At times her movement was so disrupted that she could hardly walk without stopping every two or three minutes to rest. But after visits to the family doctor and trips east to Boston's best hospitals – to meet with neurologists, cardiologists, rheumatologists, physiatrists, psychologists, psychiatrists, radiologists, infectious disease specialists, allergy specialists – and getting no definitive answers, her family felt like they had exhausted all possible avenues of medical advice and treatment. After all, there were only so many doctors they could see, just so many medications they could try, to bring Lola back to her former health. They were exhausted and felt as though they had reached out to every specialist in the world. In one meeting with a rheumatologist, they were told, 'I know something is not right, but I don't think it's physical. I don't know what it is. There's just nothing else I can do for you. I'm sorry.'

Lola had seen over 12 specialists and each had examined and worked her up thoroughly. Some had had no idea of the etiology of her condition and admitted it. Other specialists had diagnosed her with something more like fibromyalgia or non-specific autoimmune myalgia. They each initiated a different treatment protocol, yet Lola's condition did not improve. Some had even dismissed her entirely. She had almost given up any hope of finding the root cause of her disabling illness, and was even starting to question her own understanding of what was happening in her body.

As luck would have it, one of life's fortuitous coincidences arose – she was sitting alone in the dark, and absent-mindedly watching a special on the Discovery Channel called *Mystery Illness*. Every symptom described on that program she related to herself. Excitedly she shared the information with her mother. After several weeks of research and scouring the internet for more information, they finally decided to take a chance and confront one more physician, a specialist in Lyme disease. Lola returned to NYC after two years of undiagnosed debilitating illness.

Physician analysis: The self-system

Lola's case is an interesting one, where again we see a number of sustained commonalities (page 16) clearly exhibited, including: cognitive decline, the struggle between subjective and objective symptoms and her internet and media surfing for information. What interests me most about Lola's case, however, is the effect of 'the Lyme maze' on her sense of self – something that particularly concerns me due to my focus on psychiatry. In cases like Lola's, by the time patients arrive at a Lyme-literate physician, they have experienced a kind of trauma in their quest for diagnosis and treatment. And that trauma is the hidden dimension that is too often overlooked in the treatment and healing process. The recognition of this fact and careful nurturing of the 'wounded' self plays an integral part in the recovery of the tick-borne disease patient, and I think should be something all physicians are thinking about when addressing the experience of tick-borne disease. In order to investigate this issue in more depth, it will first be necessary to discuss in some detail what is meant by the terms 'self-system', 'self-concept' and 'personal identity'.

Personal identity

So, when we speak of a 'self', what is this elusive entity? Is it a convenient fiction to enable us to talk about our own uniqueness as different from others? Or is it a unique function of the human brain to encode experiences and memories in a consistent, stable, readily retrievable manner, so as to give the illusion of a unified oneness over time?

What exactly is meant by the use of the term 'self'? Children point to their body when asked that question. Obviously self does start with the body. The notion of self-hood is based upon the recognition of the physical self-model, which is found to be hard-wired and represented in the central nervous system in a particular neural network in the brain.

The area in the brain thought to be selectively engaged and involved in self-referential activity is the 'medial prefrontal cortex' (MPFC) which on brain studies (fMRI) shows this region's activity to increase as information is judged to be more self-descriptive.[55] There are also distinct neural circuits in adjacent regions which serve the cognitive and emotional aspects of self-reflection. Other research has shown that only one 'brain structure receives the prerequisite information from the sense of vision, plus information from cortical memory stores to generate a sense of "selfness".'[56] This area is the 'superior colliculus'. It has been found to receive highly precise 'retinoptic' input to the eyes, but also receive inputs from a great many other relevant areas of the cerebral cortex, vestibular inputs, auditory inputs, affective inputs, as well as information that indicates the position of the head and eyes. It is postulated that this structure allows for continuing synthesis and assessment of 'self vs. the environment'. These neural representations of a 'sense of self' are known as 'circuit impulse patterns' (CIPs) and are found to be unique to conscious experience.[57]

Moreover, the self-system is not fixed. There appears to be a stable core that is present over long stretches of time. But even the most stable core is not fixed or constant. The self and self-system are built on periods of stability and instability in response to major life events, such as illness. They obviously become more susceptible at these times to medical and psychological trauma. With negative experiences, such as failure in school, divorce, loss of job, death of a loved one, serious crippling accidents, chronic illness (such as TBD), aging and death, self-esteem obviously becomes more susceptible. The self-system, if already vulnerable, can become unstable, more vulnerable and stressed. It is not uncommon to hear patients confide: 'I feel like I am falling apart'; 'I think I am coming unglued'; 'I don't know who I am any more'; 'I've lost who I once was – I'm a shell of myself'; 'Can you help me get my old self back?'; 'When is this going to end? I feel like I'm Alice in Wonderland swirling down into a black hole and have no idea where I am going to come out'; 'I don't think I'll ever get better. I've lost all my friends and my family is tired of hearing me complain, so I don't say anything anymore. I just stuff it!'

The Lyme maze and the sense of self

Negative circumstances are expected to produce depression and lack of motivation. But negative feedback in life is an ongoing process, and healthly individuals need to be able to absorb these 'slings and arrows' and respond to them in an enlightened manner. Normally, the pre-existing 'self conceptions' of an individual support the manner in the way they wish to be treated. They dismiss what they believe to be the mistaken impressions of others.

Negative events in life are often expressed by the phrase 'stuff happens'. Healthy individuals absorb this 'stuff' and respond to it without spinning out of control. Their world does not come crashing down on them. Nor do their self-esteem and identity dissolve like a lump of sugar in hot tea. Instead, they 'become even more resolute in their convictions. They experience 'crisis' as an opportunity to evaluate their present unfavorable position and often see it as an occasion to grow stronger.

When it comes to interpersonal relationships, it is well known that an individual with a 'healthy sense of self' will dismiss mistaken impressions by others, particularly doctors. If they are told 'it is all in your head', they generally seek second and third opinions. But what happens when a person is not healthy? What happens to the sense of self for patients lost in the 'Lyme maze'?

The field of psychoneuroimmunology is devoted to the understanding of the connections between the emotional self-system, and its effect on the immune system. The self-system and one's self-esteem enter directly into the effectiveness of the immune response. Many published studies have replicated and confirmed the relationship between a perpetually negative self-image, sense of personal failure, depression, and documented reduced immunological activity.[58]

When one examines the interpersonal dynamics of tick-borne disease, it is evident that the sense of self comes under heavy assault, especially in cases like Lola's where patients experience trauma during diagnosis.

The tick-borne disease pathophysiology is a diabolical conundrum. To the patient the illness is ambiguous, threatening, mysterious, elusive, persistent and a medical anathema. Regularly a patient is faced with a wholesale dismissal of legitimate symptoms. They are unable to communicate to the physician the seriousness of their illness. 'But you don't look sick' is the common medical refrain. Often the symptoms are reframed and bundled into an impotent 'descriptive diagnosis'. Chronic fatigue syndrome, fibromyalgia, stress disorder, idiopathic peripheral neuropathy are but a few that have no etiological underpinning. The patient's intuitive sense of their body and the actual physical reality of their discomfort are medically minimized. The physical symptoms are being legitimately felt by the patient, but there can also be ambiguous cognitive or emotional subjective signals as well. They can be clear enough for the patient to conclude that 'something' is drastically wrong.

Bringing knowledge to treatment

Philip Bromberg PhD, in his excellent book *Awakening the Dreamer*, has written the following as it pertains to 'psychic trauma' and the sense of self:

> *Psychic trauma is a precipitous disruption through the invalidation of the patterns of meaning that define the experience of 'who one is'. It occurs in situations of self-invalidation that cannot be prevented or escaped from and from which there is no hope of protection, relief or soothing. If the experience is prolonged, and significant others behave as though the situation does not exist as a reality, then a state of 'autonomic hyperarousal of affect' occurs, as in post-traumatic shock disorder, that overwhelms the patient and ultimately their sanity.*

This is exactly what happens in cases like Lola's. In order to treat complex tick-borne disease cases completely, this is a 'commonality' that cannot be ignored. Physicians should make the effort to acknowledge patient trauma, and perhaps even work alongside a practicing psychiatrist or physiologist through the end of the diagnosis phase and into the treatment phase in an effort to support full patient healing.

I understand that this is not always an easy task. Tick-borne disease patients are a special class of 'walking-wounded' sufferers, victims of their undiagnosed 'invisible disability'. Their quality of life has been upended, and turned upside down. Their sense of self has been severely compromised by negative medical feedback. Just as Lola did after having been passed from doctor to doctor, these individuals feel demoralized, and are often left without hope and even without family support. Unfortunately, neuropsychiatric Lyme patients are recipients of a 'double rejection'. They are in a class by themselves.

Because of the nature of their illness, and their general frustration with the medical profession, they can be insistent, demanding and difficult. They push their doctor for an explanation of all the medical information they have researched. Some of the information is obviously of importance, obtained from journals or published articles in popular magazines. Some of the information is derived from association with other patients in self-help groups, and tick-borne disease anecdotes. Most of the time, the information is gleaned from the ubiquitous internet. A large percentage of the information brought to the physician by the patient is not very useful, and tends to be exaggerated or inaccurate. An unyielding patient can produce legitimate physician frustration, when they insist that every symptom is directly related to Lyme disease. They will cling with absolute certainty, to the belief that they are unshakably correct, and will entertain no other diagnosis for their medical condition. And more times than not, they are right.

So, instead of falling into the trap of dismissing a 'too anxious patient' for persisting in their 'Lyme obsession' or delusion, I hope we can start to reconsider the effect of this process on the patient's mental health. At this time, it is not uncommon for patients to be dropped from a practice, if they continue to argue and question their 'non-diagnosis' of 'Lyme disease', even after supposedly negative serology. Other 'encephalopathy' patients may exhibit classic psychiatric symptoms (e.g. OCD, instability, rage response, panic attack, and even bipolar episodes or frank psychotic symptoms). They appear out of place in an internal medicine practice. They are quietly classified as mentally unstable, hypochondriac or having personality disorder.

By acknowledging the effect of this condition on the sense of self, and by acknowledging the trauma associated with tick-borne disease, it is my hope that doctors can start to take a more well-rounded approach to the cases they see. The internationally respected author and practicing psychoanalyst, Michael Eagen PhD, in his book *Reshaping the Self* stated:

Every being channels myriad worlds. What makes life fascinating are the 'links' between perception, imagination, and emotion. Without this interweaving, life would be incredibly drab.

> *Nevertheless, the links between our selves and our capacities can go seriously awry. Links among perception, imagination and emotion can be wounded, warped, stunted, or severed. Our lives can tick on without us, take wrong turns, become unrecognizable. We may feel we do not fit our own body, temperament, character, personality, parents, social life, or times. We do not fit ourelves.*
>
> *For some individuals, the lack of fit between self and life is not so drastic, but still alarming. There is a nagging sense of something 'off'. Individuals may seek help in locating what feels wrong. Some need help even to admit that something* is *wrong. They ignore the 'something off' signal for as long as possible. They fear that what feels wrong will swallow them up and destroy their lives.*

This sense of dread is often a nagging, intense concern for the patient. It exists as a deep-seated fear gnawing at their sense of self. They sincerely believe they are going to die or live permanently disabled lives.

Psychoneuroimmunology and the 'self' system

The physician treating the patient with TBD must be aware that many patients are suffering not only from the physical symptoms of the syndrome, but also from a 'wounded' self-system and personal 'identity'. Psychic and emotional trauma, which are a result of the negative experiences of being misdiagnosed, are detrimental to the patient's healing capacity and to the strength of their immune response. Life stressors arising from the illness, like loss of an important relationship, can inflict grave wounds on the self-system. One of the defense systems of the psyche is known as 'dissociation', and this psychological state has been shown to be responsible for compromised immune activity and lowered NK function. Such negative statements as:

- I'll never get better
- I go around and around in circles
- I feel completely worthless

- I'm not good to anyone anymore
- I'm just a burden to my family
- If I have to live this way, what's the point?
- Nobody believes how sick I am
- They all say 'But you don't look sick'
- I feel like I am standing outside my life and looking at it through a glass wall.

are the cries of a wounded self system.

The self-system, a sense of wellbeing and a solid personal identity should be considered as essential for healing. The treating physician needs to be aware of this sensitive neurological network and direct his/her attention toward it, as if it were another critical organ system, crucial to the health and recovery of the TBD patient. The physician prescribes antibiotics, herbals, nutrients and other pharmaceutical and physical treatments to overcome the disease. The same dedication and care must also be taken to treat a compromised 'self-system', which can.be looked upon as a 'psychic healing center'. Empathic, one-on-one, half-hour to one-hour visits, preferably no more than six weeks apart at the outset, are the backbone of treatment, to my mind, and one of the key factors in the patient overcoming his/her illness.

Martin Buber in his classic book *I and Thou,* discusses what he calls an 'authentic encounter with another' and the difference between 'real meeting' and 'mis-meeting'. The authentic experience of 'hearing' and 'being heard' is what Buber would call the 'real meeting' which in my practise creates a 'healing medical dialogue' and a bond of trust with the TBD patient. This encounter should not be minimized and relegated to simple formula history taking (mis-meeting), because it is through this process that a vital 'healing relationship' is established. In this encounter, the patient's self-system is validated, often for the first time, and liberated from the hidden shame of having an undiagnosed illness.

'I feel like the weight of the world has been lifted from my shoulders. It all makes sense to me now. And I don't care how long it takes me to get well. Just knowing that I'm not crazy and you were a doctor who really listened to me for the first time, that means everything to me.'

The patient no longer feels demoralized by his/her illness. Nor does s/he feel crazy, malingering, hypochondriacal, or like an unpopular medical pest. The physician's 'meeting' must engage with the 'dissociated self system' and injured personal identity. This renewed 'psychic self centre' quite possibly holds the key to the ultimate success or failure of treatment.

Chapter 10

Kate Vance, age 34 The family-system response to tick-borne disease

Kate and Dylan had been married for two years. For a year and a half everything had been bliss. People said that they were perfect for each other. They were the quintessential special couple. They both seemed to intuit each other's needs.

They had lived in New York City for six months, having moved to the 'Big Apple' from Scranton, Pennsylvania. They were new to everything in the city and they loved it! Trying new restaurants, seeing Broadway shows, running in Central Park, and of course shopping. Kate had accepted a job with a prestigious law firm in the city, down on Wall Street. She had graduated first in her class at University of Pennsylvania School of Law and was honored to be at the top of her class. Her reputation preceded her, and she was welcomed by the firm with open arms and even given a prestigious corner window. Kate was excited, enthusiastic and adapted to the new environment at work easily. Her first two cases, which she litigated, were very successful. 'Easier than law school,' she had commented to her husband at breakfast. She made new friends quickly and was immediately accepted by her colleagues.

Then the strange changes began. At first, they were subtle and barely noticeable. Things at home started to change imperceptibly. Her activities diminished. She wasn't as enthusiastic about going out at night after work. In fact, her appetite was 'off' and new restaurants didn't hold the same appeal. Her physical energy seemed to wane and she stopped running in the park. She reduced her Pilates classes down to once a week and didn't seem to get the same pleasure from them as before. Her muscles hurt more after her work-outs and this continued into the next day. She had Dylan rub them for a half hour or so after she got home. From time to time, she found herself taking deep breaths, and just needing more air. For the first time, she noticed she was going to bed much earlier, but not sleeping as well. And though she was loath to admit it, she found herself ignoring amorous hints from Dylan, which she had previously welcomed.

Kate was heartsick that her libido had fled the scene. A year before, it had used to be equal to her husband's, but lately it had completely disappeared. She was constantly tired, depressed and felt no enthusiasm at all for making love. A little snuggling with Dylan at night in bed was all she could muster. The bedroom for her had become a place to crash out exhausted. She just wanted to shut the world out, nothing more.

Then other things in their relationship began to change. At first, almost imperceptibly. Dylan began to get under her skin. It was just little incidents, like the time he carelessly left the milk out of the fridge, and spilled orange juice on the counter that he didn't clean up after himself. Or the time he was running out of the apartment for a meeting, and forgot to pick up his underwear and socks off the bedroom floor. She didn't say anything at first, biting her lip, taking a deep breath, and counting to 10. But after a few more trivial annoyances, her anger against Dylan began to escalate.

Suddenly, one Saturday morning when they were cleaning the apartment together, Dylan knocked over a flower vase with his broom. She exploded. She was shocked at the intensity of her outburst. This kind of behavior had never occurred before and she was mortified. It happened again two weeks later over a TV channel preference. Dylan chose Monday night football over her preference of the Voice. When Dylan switched the channel, she went ballistic and hurled the remote control at his head, missing him by inches.

Chapter !0

Kate's unreasonable behaviors continued. She was like a hungry snapping turtle. No matter what Dylan tried to do to please her, it just didn't seem to be enough. After another of what had become regular outbursts, Dylan hugged her and said, 'Honey, why are you being so crazy? I don 't get it. What am I doing wrong?'

'I don 't know what 's happening to me,' she said tearfully. 'I don't seem to have any self-control anymore. Just about everything annoys the hell out of me.'

She was totally confused by her own behavior. Kate knew she wasn't herself, but it seemed she couldn't do anything about it. Try as she might to be more in control of her emotions, her mood still fluctuated almost daily.

And it wasn't just Dylan who kept setting her off. She was less sociable and more irritable at work as well. On one occasion, she left another attorney's office in tears. It was only a minor disagreement over how to handle a client's appeal to a higher court. Kate took it personally as a rejection of her legal ability and felt humiliated.

Just about everything bothered her. All of her senses seemed to be exaggerated. The florescent lights at work felt far too bright, as did the sunlight outdoors; both gave her a splitting headache.

The copier toner smell made her nauseated and the background music almost drove her crazy. She began wearing dark glasses everywhere outside as well as at work when she was alone. She bought herself a pair of Bose headphones to block out the extraneous grating sounds of the city. The sound of an ambulance or a fire truck made her cringe with pain and almost brought tears to her eyes.

Her headaches, which had been rare before, became regular and unbearable It was like a blinding pressure as if her head was caught in a vice. She hardly recognized herself anymore. No matter what Dylan tried to do to help her, she declined his suggestions and efforts. This included going out with friends, going to the gym, trying a new restaurant. But nothing made her feel better. She was emotionally flat, and just wanted to be left alone and disappear.

Kate had tried initially to get some medical answers. She went to see her new family doctor, Dr Brenda Wilson, who spent extra time with her and took what Kate thought was an ocean of blood samples. Everything from the laboratory analysis came back letter perfect, as reported by Dr Wilson with a knowing smile at their next meeting.

'More normal than normal,' her doctor said.

'Even my hormones? They feel like they've been put in a blender and chopped up,' Kate said, incredulously.

'You 're fine, Kate,' the doctor said, 'Just stressed. Believe me. This city will grind you up and spit you out if you're not careful. You're trying to do too much. Slow down. Maybe it would help to talk to someone. Sounds like your marriage could use a little fine tuning.'

Shortly after the visit, Kate and Dylan had a consultation with a psychologist, Marion Dixon PhD, who after three sessions pronounced their marriage healthy. 'Simple early marital adjustment problems. Nothing more. Nothing serious,' she diagnosed. She did suggest Kate see a psychiatrist for what appeared to be depression.

During Kate's first visit to Dr Ronald Ferbune on the Upper West Side of Manhattan she admitted to a number of other symptoms, including persistent insomnia that had been occurring for three months. She would fall on her bed exhausted, but sleep refused to come to her.

'I feel like I haven't slept a single minute all night. But the worst symptom I have,' she admitted to him, 'is the sensation of being cut off from the world. It's like I'm there and not there. I'm looking at myself interacting in the world, but I'm outside myself looking in. I feel completely insane.'

Reluctantly, after some resistance to the idea of medication for her symptoms, she accepted a prescription for a pain killer, an antidepressant and sleeping medication for insomnia. A month or so into the medicine, she had to admit that she did feel a little better.

She was more in control and not as emotional. But she still felt flat. No sparkle. No sense of excitement. No libido. She constantly lamented that she just wanted her former life back. Nothing more than that.

As things seemed to normalize, she told people she was fine even when she knew she was not. She learned to control her rage and let her flat, weak energy become normal. But months passed and she started to disengage from herself. It was almost as if she wasn't in her body anymore, but watching her life on a movie screen as she went through the motions of every day.

When she told Dylan about this kind of depersonalization she was feeling every day, he insisted she take a trip to see a new psychiatrist. She wasn't progressing enough. Things weren't getting better in the way they were supposed to.

During her first visit with the new doctor, as she was recounting her history she heard herself describing symptoms that she had come to know as normal. Things like consistent itching, and weird arm twitches, and waking up in the night drenched in sweat after a nightmare – these had all become part of the routine she had learned to accept. This was her new normal.

But as she recounted her day-to-day experience to her new psychiatrist, she realized the doctor seemed alarmed. The doctor suspected there was some organic route to these other symptoms that needed to be addressed. With a proper diagnosis and proper treatment, Kate might be able to make a full recovery.

Physician analysis: The family system

In Kate's case, the effect of her illness on her family and relatives is almost as debilitating to her as the illness itself. Without a proper diagnosis, she is stuck in a devastating cycle of damage to her relationship that is difficult to break free from.

In an acute health crisis or emergency (those that resolve in days, weeks or even months) good 'technical biomedical' care takes priority. There is almost always a predictable time frame, with a more or less predictable outcome. Patients endure the inevitable hardships for a defined period of time. Their family members usually are supportive in the crisis (emergency room visits for kidney stones, for example, bronchial pneumonia, broken bones or appendicitis). But when symptoms persist and progress, sometimes for years without answers, we start to see a breakdown of that system.

Most doctors do not consider the effect of this Lyme maze on caregivers and family. The individual should not be considered in isolation, but rather as an integral part of a dynamic 'family care giving system'. The total family system, and not just the individual patient in isolation, becomes the central focus in a chronic tick-borne illness.

Some of the questions often asked by the family of someone with a tick-borne disease include:

> 'What is normal family coping?'
>
> 'How should we as family members adapt to living with illness?'
>
> 'What can we expect, over time and well into the future? Is the patient able to be cured?'
>
> 'What is a remission?'
>
> 'What is a relapse?'

These are questions that can go unanswered for years.

This delay can be especially frustrating in cases of Lyme and other tick-borne disease as so many wrong pathways may be followed in the mean time. As we see in Kate's case, and in Lola's (Chapter 9), the effect of this infection on the mind seriously complicates the experience of the patient.

Chapter 10

Tick-borne disease and the mind/body dichotomy

Tick-borne diseases, in addition to their difficult and mixed development (making diagnosis and treatment extremely difficult), have another inherent problem for the patient and their physicians. They must overcome together, the medical dilemma inherent in the 'mind / body' dichotomy. This is recognized as the 'infamous' split between our subjective 'consciousness' and the 'material reality' of our physical body.

Unfortunately, the concept of 'mind' or 'consciousness' has long been treated independently of our physical 'bodies'. Modern medicine has practically ignored the critical relationship of the 'metaphysical' mind to the physical body. Instead it has concentrated mostly on the 'physical brain', as it relates to its physical body. The usefulness of the subjective experience, by most current standards, is seen as being extremely limited, when applied to the area of clinical diagnosis and treatment. In fact, most overworked physicians consider 'mind', or subjective symptoms, to be a liability in the effectivenees of their treatment protocols (outside of psychiatry). For them, the fewer the subjective complaints that their patients have (or admit to), the more compliant and cooperative those patients are considered to be. 'Mind' only becomes important to the contemporary physician when it is recognized as an extension of our 'hardwired' neurobiology.

This mysterious, vascularized, gray-and-white-matter mass of spongy synapses has intrigued and captured the interest of research medicine for many years. As early as 1990, the Society for Neuroscience designated the subsequent 10 years as the 'Decade of the Brain'. Since that time the organization has grown from a handful of scientists to over 25,000 members.[59]

Sophisticated neuro-imaging techniques (MRI, SPECT scan, PET scan), biochemical neurotransmitter analysis, genetic investigations of gene-driven mental illness, brain peptide production and single-cell-evoked potential probes, and stem cell brain repair, have allowed researchers to better understand the brain's previously inaccessible neurological secrets, but we still have a long way to go. Computer algorithims for medical diagnosis have strongly influenced the field of diagnosis and treatment of brain diseases. Medicine has become more and more reliant on sophisticated technology. Robotic surgery, the suject of science fiction a mere 25 years ago, is an everyday occurrence in operating rooms today. But TBD seems ironically to be left out of the technological revolution in medicine, because laboratory technology has not yet caught up with the complexity of the illness. Or at least more sophisticated testing methods are not utilized even though they now exist.

The treating physician and a patient's emotional health

The patient's own belief systems about health and illness are critical to the treatment outcome of any condition. For discussion purposes, I view tick-borne disease as not just localized in one organ, or even multiple organ systems in a solitary, infected patient. The useful working disease definition should be understood as a 'tick-borne family illness system'. The physician needs to join the 'family illness system' to create a therapeutic alliance in the best interests of the patient.

Naturally, the processes of the disease strongly influence both patient and family responses. Chronic, persistent and relapsing, tick-borne disease inserts itself into family life with a vengeance. It affects the life not only of the individual infected patient, but also of other members of the family who must adapt continually to radical changes in the ill person. The age of the patient, the developmental tasks appropriate for that person, and the stage of the family life cycle, all contribute to defining the strengths and weaknesses of the family support system.

We have seen these strengths and weaknesses fluctuate

throughout all of the presented cases. Alex's family system was of course affected by his struggle in school, and his emotional and angry outbursts. Sarah's family had to change their entire routine and rhythm to accommodate their mother's condition, before even realizing what it actually was. Tick-borne disease affects a much larger network or system than just the infected patient, and it is important for physicians and patients alike to carry this understanding with them through their journey.

An unwelcome family member

In a somewhat analogous way, the appearance of chronic tick-borne disease in a family partially resembles the addition of a new, but unwelcome, family member, which also requires high cohesion and maintenance. If the illness coincides with the 'autonomous' stage of family life, it can cause serious problems. The 'sickness' demands of borreliosis (Lyme) for 'cohesion' and nurturing are in conflict with the high-energy demands of autonomy and independence. For example, when a parent develops a chronic tick-borne disease during the child-rearing phase of care taking, the family is severely taxed.

For each family member exposed to tick-borne disease, the course of his or her illness and treatment may be completely different in comparison one with another. This depends on the length of time a family member has had the illness, the degree of their disability, the medications used and the routes of administration; the acute symptoms, or persistence of symptoms, may all be manifested at the same time. The result is that the family is continually being placed under tremendous interpersonal, psychological and physical stress.

Economic stress also adds to the family's load. Costs for treatment can run exceptionally high, particularly if long-term IV therapy is necessary, and in the US the bias against Lyme disease by most insurance companies often results in the patient being totally responsible for the cost of treatment.[60] In the UK, the problem is the NHS's unwillingness to recognize that Lyme can be a chronic problem.

This unremitting stress cuts deeply into the wellbeing of the family. Unfortunately, the chronic stress also exacerbates the Lyme symptoms of each family member and prolongs their illness.[61]

It should be noted that each family member experiences his or her own 'life crisis' outside the family system as well as inside it. This leads to differences in the severity of impact to the family system as a whole (father's or mother's work to support the family vs. child's academic success and school attendance) and creates different family stresses, which are unique to each individual.

Clearly, 'fatigue, exhaustion and insomnia' in a child who can't attend school will have different consequences and a different impact on a family, than in a father or mother who is the family breadwinner. Although they have similar symptoms, the child is usually supported by a network of services and attended by the school system. A parent who is too sick to go to work, or perform adequately in his/her job, is in danger of losing the critical economic support that his/her family depends on. A parent responsible for childcare, on the other hand, who is severely symptomatic and handicapped, does not have the capacity to be responsible for the household and the care of the children. In this instance, the whole nurturing system of the family falls into a state of disrepair.

The extent to which a 'chronically ill family system' is either supported or divided by their extended family system, obviously affects the outcome and the stress experienced by all members of the family-illness system.

This concept of 'systems thinking' is relevant at every level in the approach we take to Lyme. We can look at the micro level, exploring the bacterium and its behaviors, or at a bigger level in considering the effect of disease on the individual, or the family system, or the medical system, or ultimately on the whole population.

Chapter 10

The following sections of this book will start to explore Lyme and tick-borne disease in the context of bigger systems thinking, and how this thinking differs from country to country around the world.

Part Three

Gregory Bateson, spirochetes and general systems linkages

Chapter 11

The legacy of Gregory Bateson

Gregory Bateson, the famous English anthropologist who made his home in California, has been an inspiration throughout my lifetime. He stands as one of the intellectual giants in the pantheon of 20th-century thinkers. Bateson was blessed and cursed with a mind that saw through the superficiality of things into a world of pattern and form which 'lay beyond the norm'. He was my professor at Stanford and my research director for my psychiatric residency in Hawaii. He was a charismatic six foot five, rumpled, spell-binding lecturer who rarely used notes or a written syllabus. Whether he spoke in front of a small class. or a packed 700-seat amphitheater, he spoke spontaneously, seeming to make his presentation an effortless conversation with his audience. He never seemed to start at the beginning, but rather to randomly begin somewhere in the middle of a complicated thought. Listening to him, one got the sense that it was a journey of discovery through a labyrinth to reach a central point. He seemed to think through an issue out loud, raising more questions than answers to a particular topic, on a myriad of subjects.

At Stanford, I attended his postgraduate lectures on communication theory (he had recently authored the famous research with Don Jackson MD on the double-bind theory in schizophrenia), cybernetics, information theory, general systems theory and cultural anthropology. I remember many times after being mesmerized by a two-hour lecture class with Bateson, I would leave the class befuddled. I knew I had spent two hours listening to something important, but damned if I understood what it was exactly about.

For the purposes of this book I will attempt to integrate some of Bateson's central ideas, particularly his general systems theory, with the TBD pandemic.

I personally try to use 'general systems theory' thinking in my TBD medical practice. This approach helps me to understand the complicated interactions of TBD at all levels. This way of thinking has had an enormous effect on how I view TBD. The teachings and personal contact with Gregory Bateson have influenced how I think about this highly controversial and complicated disease entity.

Gregory Bateson regularly explored and spoke eloquently about this type of thinking throughout his career. He argued that living systems make up the biosphere, and that these living systems should be looked upon as 'mental processes' in the metaphorical sense. A world of 'Mind' is how Bateson would describe it. One particular form of 'Mind' is human consciousness with its survival advantages. Such attributes as language, writing, mathematical ability, invention and now rampant technology with AI, have conferred on the human species distinct evolutionary assets.

However, these assets carry with them serious consequences for the planet. They have their dark side. Bateson warned that these characteristics lead to a distinct isolation from the natural processes of evolution. Self-seeking 'conscious purposefulness' has become 'a pathology'.

What mattered to Bateson was the relational connection between man and nature. For example, there is an inter-related dependency between a forest ecosystem and the questing of the tick population. Add the gypsy moth to the linkage, and the relationship between the gypsy moth and the forest devastation it can produce becomes significant for the tick population and human disease. With gypsy moth forest infestation, there will be a corresponding loss of oak trees and with this a significant loss of acorn production. It is well known that smaller mammals as well as deer feed on these acorns. With less food supply there is a reduction in the general population of small host mammals, including the most prolific host carriers – namely, the white-footed mice. Fewer animal hosts will determine the subsequent reduction in numbers of ticks, by virtue of the fact that ticks go through a metamorphosis from eggs laid by the adult female, to a feeding larva, then to a feeding nymph and finally to a sexually mature adult female tick, with each stage of the tick life cycle needing a sustaining blood meal from a mammalian host in order to survive. A diminished population of infected white-footed mice thus leads to a less infected human population.

There was no question for Bateson but that humans were inseparable from, and enmeshed in, the world-mind-system. And their special characteristic of conscious purposefulness too often was 'making a mess of things' in the delicately balanced biosphere.

If I expand my intellectual vision, I move from the structural anatomy of the Borrelia spirochete itself, to contemplate the way this bacterium is integrated into a complex ecosystem, in which humans have become an unsuspecting host. The bacterium itself creates a complex disease state that affects all the physiological systems of the body. It creates a foreign sensation in the psyche of patients that alerts them to the fact that something is terribly askew with their health. This takes place in the larger context of their family and their medical support systems. This in turn affects the administration and the oversight played by different political concerns (medical societies, insurance standards for reimbursement, pharmaceutical companies and government oversight at local, state and federal levels). As the general systems model expands outward, we see it encompassing countries and continents reaching World Health and United Nations concerns.

Bateson's focus on hierarchical levels of an integrated system applies directly to the understanding of tick-borne disease. It encompasses general systems theory, evolutionary biology, cybernetics, anthropology and other specialties.

Bateson often said, metaphor is one of the most effective tools for representing and describing aspects of the world, but it is obviously not the world. When one investigates complex wholes, metaphor can allow for a more effective way of understanding the relationships within a system, sometimes even more effectively than scientific or rational descriptive analysis. 'All you can do is point at the object and just stand there. That's it. That's as close as you will get to the "reality" of it. Your words are only the map, not the object, not the territory!'; 'What you say it is, is not it.'

Defining the territory

Though the incident I am about to recount occurred more than 58 years ago, it has relevance to the TBD controversy today.

When I was a medical student I was captain of the University of Toronto debating team. We were given the opportunity to debate Oxford University. Oxford was to choose the topic and pick the side of the argument they wished to defend. They chose the following and to defend the affirmative position: 'Resolved that since birth control is contrary to natural law, it follows that "contraception" should be abolished'. We were left with the opposing side, and that was to defend contraception. We confidently embraced our side of the argument; the science was indisputable.

There were three Oxford debaters who arrived to debate us: a carrot-topped, freckled debater who looked no more than 14; a plump, overweight, sweaty, flushed, cherubic-looking fellow; and finally the captain. He was elegant and carried himself like he knew it.

I sincerely believed that the facts were indisputably on our sides. After all I was a medical student and birth control and contraception were obviously necessities in the modern world. There were the factual concerns of population explosion. There were the realities of world famine, scarcity of resources, high infant mortality, deaths of women forced to abort with no medical care, communicable STDs (no AIDS at that time but plenty of others), on and on. We thought that all we needed to do was stick to the obvious facts and it would be a cake walk. Victory was assured.

We presented our case well and articulately. Facts were clearly stated. Even some dramatic case highlights. But the 'Brits' didn't debate our facts. They didn't need to do so. They didn't need facts. They had superior language skills. It was a clear case of style and persuasion over facts and substance. It was their map. They defined the territory. We had no other recourse but to try and maneuver within it. But of course, on that 'ground' we were no match for their superior command of the English language. We were roundly defeated.

I never forgot that lesson. And I think it applicable to the whole TBD controversy. Over and over again 'opinion' passing for evidence-based science in the form of outdated and inaccurate guidelines, with vital research information excluded from consideration, continues to be preached as the standard of care. Opinions by so-called experts are not neutral clinical science. They are biased and based often on financial self-interest.

From my 35 years of clinical practice with TBD, the issue of persistent spirochetal infection before and after treatment, in multiple organ systems (muscles, joints, energy system, nervous system), has been scientifically researched and proven beyond a doubt. The impact of the co-infections on the pathogenesis of borreliosis is a complex synergistic tangle manifesting itself over years in different organ systems. Often four or more intracellular organisms (see Chapter 4) contribute to the patient's chronic and unrelenting symptom presentation. A vast research literature exists, detailing the persistence of TBD infections. Why is the mantra of 'no scientific evidence' of chronicity repeated in the IDSA guidelines *ad nauseam*? The infamous statement that appeared in the IDSA and CDC guidelines stands alone as a monument to dishonest, non-scientific, self-serving, ignorant, politically biased dogma.

> *To date there is no convincing biological evidence for the existence of symptomatic, chronic* B. burgdorferi *infection among patients after receipt of the recommended treatment regimens for Lyme. Antibiotic therapy has not proven to be useful and is not recommended for patients with chronic (6 months or more) subjective symptoms after administration of recommended treatment regimens for Lyme disease.*

Of equal importance is the statement issued by the attorney general of Connecticut in May 2008:

> *My office uncovered undisclosed financial interests held by several of the most powerful IDSA guideline panelists. This panel improperly ignored or minimized consideration of alternative medical opinion and evidence regarding chronic Lyme disease, potentially raising serious questions whether the recommendations reflected all the relevant science.*

Back to the lesson of the debate – if you limit the territory of what is defined as a TBD patient, you define the boundaries of the scientific debate. If you restrict the boundaries, you can limit access to the territory. If you limit access to the territory, you restrict the understanding of the true nature of the illness. By declaring persistent TBD to be a non-existent, scientifically unproven condition, you restrict treatment to certain minimal interventions, with the result that patients wander blindly through a medical labyrinth.

What then is the real 'territory'? How are we to define it?

If Borrelia alone is defined only as a spiral, fixed and unchangeable bacterial form, every other form visualized under the microscope is considered irrelevant. This includes the cystic forms, delineated, photographed and published, as well as the L-forms (cell-wall-deficient forms) and plasmids. Deny the existence of these forms, then the issue of 'persisters' no longer becomes an area of scientific inquiry. Most infectious disease specialists have not acknowledged the fact of their existence. And if they have admitted that 'there is something there', they have also declared that they have no impact on treatment. By eliminating these stealth forms from the equation, they preclude the likelihood of survival, relapse and persistence after 'adequate treatment'. In the words of one infamous infectious disease specialist, 'The whole notion is nothing more than science fiction.'

On the other hand, if the territory accepts these forms as relevant, new areas of research can be opened, and the phenomenon of resistance and relapse can be better understood.

To deny that the 'cyst forms' are a serious biological protective response to an environmental threat to the spiral form, is rather like studying the caterpillar in isolation from the 'metamorphosis' cycle that ultimately produces the brilliantly winged monarch butterfly. To understand the butterfly, you must follow its precisely mapped and coded migration pattern, over thousands of miles, to one particular location in Mexico. By limiting the study to the crawling caterpillar only, the majestic monarch never emerges from its chrysalis.

Enter back into the debate, the late esteemed English anthropologist Gregory Bateson. As I have said, he believed strongly in the scientific validity and explanatory value of 'general systems theory'. He argued that a system (a system being defined as a community of interacting parts, mutually interdependent, communicating at various levels of a hierarchy in both directions directly through a balanced flow of information) could exhibit properties of 'mind or purposefulness'. He illustrated this radical concept with examples in nature. He further maintained that these complex systems were exhibiting properties of 'consciousness'.

Building a dialogue

Mary Catherine Bateson, Bateson's oldest daughter, used a type of literary form in her writings about her father's ideas that she called a 'metalogue'. With this method, she was able to fictionalize a type of 'dialogue' between herself and her father that explained many of his difficult abstract concepts. This search for insight into a complex subject was the basis of her 'metalogues'.

I would like to use the format of Mary Catherine Bateson's metalogue to convey some of Gregory Bateson's ideas that are hyper-relevant to tick-borne disease.

The metalogue

Raxlen: Gregory, today I'd like to talk to you about ticks and Lyme disease – not the most entertaining of subjects. I suspect that this topic falls under the heading of 'mind-in-process and the effects of conscious purpose on human adaptation'.

Bateson: Yes, my thoughts on the issue were published in a book entitled *Our Own Metaphor*, by my daughter, Mary Catherine Bateson. The insights gained at that conference have held true to this day and are not irrelevant in the modern world. In fact, those insights are more relevant than ever. Look around, Bernard. We are despoiling our environment, our rainforests, our oceans, and feeding climate change, with the disappearance of 50 per cent of our coral reefs.

Half the world – over three billion people – live below the poverty line with significantly reduced life expectancy. We have nuclear stand-offs with unstable leaders, paranoid fingers on the trigger; a possible nuclear disaster waiting to happen; infant mortality worldwide still unbelievably high, for all our medical miracles; and less and less biodiversity, with endangered species disappearing at an alarming rate.

Mind in nature has become fundamentally deranged! Our disconnected 'minds' are divorced from the natural world. We are 'thinking' ourselves into oblivion.

Raxlen: These are certainly scary times. And I think a lot about the way that our effect on the planet is influencing the Lyme world. But before we get to that, I know you believe that unless we approach something equivalent to the concept of mind-in-nature, and a sense of the 'sacred' as opposed to the 'profane' (ignorance of interdependent connections that sustain the fragile web of life) we can never achieve 'Grace'.

Gregory, what do you mean exactly by this term? Sorry, it's a lovely word but I don't quite understand how you are using it.

Bateson: If I had to define it – and I don't want to, since it is a unique feeling state – I'd start off by saying you either achieve it or you don't. I suppose it could be understood as a state of being where the relationships between things are looked upon as a linked processes contained within a hierarchy of increasingly complex systems, all with varying degrees of interdependence.

For human beings, for example, you could say Grace begins with 'molecules that form cellular structures, that are organized into interdependent organ systems, that constitute the unique individual, whose life is interdependent with his nuclear and extended family, who themselves are part of a community neighborhood, which is interdependent with the town or city of which it is part, that is interdependent with the state and country and finally the continent and planet.' In other words, everything is connected – and those connections are healthy and functional.

Raxlen: I've heard you speak to the point that the very survival of 'mankind' is predicated on understanding these linkages.

Bateson: Probably a bit overstated, but not far from the truth!

Raxlen: I'd like to understand the Lyme disease epidemic using your insights. I'm not quite sure how to apply it though.

Bateson: I think I know what you're after. But I want to change the discussion briefly, from ticks and spirochetes to cats and rabbits.

Raxlen: Sounds like another metaphor.

Bateson: Not really; this is just an illustrative example of 'planning and problem solving' gone haywire. Good intentions, problem-solving strategies, and conscious purpose may be there, but misunderstanding of the system produces exactly the opposite of the desired effects.

Raxlen: Yes, I'd like to hear about it and see if there is some parallel to tick-borne disease. It sounds similar to a plan to eliminate deer to wipe out spirochetes.

Bateson: Something like that. In his book *Lyme Disease: The Ecology of a Complex System*, Richard Ostfeld has described an island between New Zealand and Antarctica which was home to a unique endemic parakeet and an endemic real bird, as well as a lot of penguins and sea birds of various types. In the 19th century the island was colonized by 'sealers' who were isolated from their families and loved ones for an interminable length of time. So, they decided that they needed the companionship of more than each other. As a result, they brought in pet cats, and a ready source of food – rabbits!

Raxlen: There were no other predators?

Bateson: No predators; only rabbits hopping around all over the place. In fact, by the end of the 20th century on a 34-kilometer-long island they grew to a population of 130,000 rabbits and their grazing eradicated all of the vegetation. So, to solve the problem, they needed to get rid of the rabbits. Those involved in wishing to maintain a balanced ecology used a deadly flea-transmitted virus called a 'myxoma virus' that killed rabbits. Once the rabbits were gone, the hungry cats attacked the nesting sea birds for food, and practically eliminated them. And of course, the island population desperately wanted the seabirds back. So, what do you think happened?

Raxlen: The islanders killed the cats. Did that finally solve the problem?

Bateson: Not really. With the eradication of the cats, there was another rabbit explosion. This couldn't be controlled by the myxoma virus, because the rabbits became resistant. Satellite images of the island started to show rapid defoliation. And without vegetation, the sea birds (which were now protected) had no nesting sites. No birds' eggs, no birds.

Raxlen: You would think at the outset the whole idea of ecological restoration of the island was a solid idea, in keeping with the principles of modern ecological thinking. So why did it go so wrong? What should have been done? Just sit back and watch the island implode and die?

Bateson: The problem isn't that one 'should' or 'shouldn't' intervene in the system, but a better understanding of the system is necessary so that unforeseen consequences don't happen, You get some idea of how good intentions can go off in all directions. I sense that Lyme disease is a far more intricately complicated problem than rabbits and cats, though the thinking may still apply. There are innumerable variables that make this complex bio-ecosystem of bacterial infection, insect-vector 'tick' transmission, human/ mammalian hosts, changes in biodiversity, susceptible suburban residences, over-population of white-footed mice (the main US Borrelia reservoir) and deer, and medical/ political resistance to the epidemic.

As Ostfeld has written, 'Infectious diseases are ecological systems. Interactions among organisms determine disease risk. Once the pathogen has been identified, we must cast a broader net to identify where in nature the pathogen comes from, what regulates its abundance and distribution, and what influences and what regulates its contact rate with its hosts, including humans.'

I can imagine a hierarchical system, where the levels all influence and connect to each other. This would include the smallest pieces of the system (like molecules and bacteria) and would expand to higher levels of the system (like towns and institutions). Along every step of the way, each level, from human to family, to neighborhood to government, would influence the others.

All of these systems are linked together with information that arises from the top down as well as from the bottom up, which constitutes a unified whole.

Raxlen: Is this how I should think about this problem?

Bateson: It might help you get a better understanding of Lyme disease (that is, tick-borne disease) and the problems associated with it. If you investigate the errors of 'thinking' inherent in the system, you can find bigger problems affecting the patient. For example, a seemingly small error in any part of the system can lead to catastrophic ramifications for a patient's health.

Raxlen: So, by understanding the errors in thinking, I can better grasp those issues that make this subject so contentious?

Bateson: I would say so. And the first error in thinking that stands out to me is the name given to the disease. It might as well be called 'tangerine' disease.

Raxlen: It's called 'Lyme' disease after a town in Connecticut where it was first uncovered.

Bateson: There is much power in a name, Bernard. Naming things correctly gives them a particular reality. So, may I humbly suggest that we follow a more formal classification, so that my father William Bateson won't haunt me at nights lecturing me as to the importance of Linnaeus classification? Let's give it the dignity of its full name:

Kingdom – Prokaryote (bacteria)
Division – Gracilicutes (bacteria with thin cell walls)
Class – Scotobacteria (bacteria that do not use light for energy)
Order – Spirochaeteles (bacteria that are spiral)
Family – Spirochaetaceae (spirochetes with particular cell characteristics)
Genus – Borrelia (a group of tick-borne spirochetes discovered a century ago by the bacteriologist Amedee Borrel)
Species – Burgdorferi (after Willie Burgdorfer)

Raxlen: But why go to all that trouble? Lyme disease seems so much easier to understand.

Bateson: Yes, but the name of this complicated disease syndrome designated as Lyme tells us nothing about the bacterial specifics. The name instead brings forth overwhelming and misleading emotional hysteria. And at the same time tells us nothing at all about the actual characteristics of the bacterium itself. The naming of it 'Lyme' moves from bacterial science to fantasy. Then everything and nothing can be attributed to the name at the same time, depending on what side of the fence you're on.

Raxlen: That's okay with me. But I'm not clear on what you mean by the disease being 'a hierarchically linked system of intricately linked subsystems'. When you talk like that it makes my head spin…

Bateson: Let's look at the problem not as a single bacterial spirochete causing illness, but as a more complicated systems problem.

Raxlen: Well then, let's start by defining what you mean by system.

Bateson: There are some key concepts when thinking about a system.

1. The whole is greater than the sum of its parts.
2. The system is defined by 'boundaries'.
3. The system exhibits homeostasis – it seeks stability, but must adapt and change to remain stable. Changes come about as a result of the reception of new information.
4. The behavior of the individual units within the system can only be understood with reference to the system to which they are connected.
5. There are two types of system: 'open' and 'closed'. An open system receives input from the environment and has a dynamic interaction with it. Since I understand from you that we are really talking about more than one bacterium (*Borrelia burgdorferi*) that together give you what is loosely called 'Lyme disease', we are looking at a multi-microbial , multi-infectious, multi-systemic entity, are we not?

Raxlen: Yes, we certainly are. I like the term 'tick-borne disease' – that way you are not limited to one organism. Then, by definition, the clinical presentation has to change as well, if you have this mixed bacterial population. Complexity as well as clarity can happen at the same time.

Bateson: If we look at the study of tick-borne disease as an interacting system, it might look something like a ladder of ascending complexity, each hierarchically related rung contributing to the understanding of tick-borne disease, and also making clearer why the system in part may have areas of 'closed input' which limit the system's stability and adaptability.

Raxlen: Sounds very dense to me. I think I understand the ideas of open and closed systems, but I find it hard to understand how to apply it.

Bateson: Alright, let's start with the skeletal frame of the system and elaborate from there. The following is the order of hierarchically organized levels of complexity:

Raxlen: No cats or rabbits?

Bateson: Not this time. Not in the same way. But we can't forget them, not just yet anyway. If you are going to build a general system's model for Lyme disease, aka tick-borne disease, you need at the very minimum to identify interacting units through which information flows unobstructed in both directions; these are known as feedback loops. An axiom of general systems thinking is that the behavior of individual units can be 'understood' only in the context of the system to which they belong.

Raxlen: You mean to say the whole is greater than the sum of its parts?

Bateson: Exactly; that is one of the first fundamentals in my previous definition of a system.

Raxlen: Anything else I need to know about systems?

Bateson: Not really. Not for our purposes. But there is a vast literature on general systems theory and its application to multiple disciplines, from guided missiles to an intricate, delicately balanced ecosystem in a thriving forest. For example, a certain bacterium carried in the gut of a termite is necessary for the insect to digest wood fiber from decaying fallen trees, which leads to the regular renewal of nutrients in the soil and the subsequent sustainability of the forest. This small bacterium takes us from debris (dead wood) to living plants.

Raxlen: Are there any other first principles which I should be aware of? My head hurts.

Bateson: Let's just say for the purposes of our discussion, and not to overwhelm you, it's important to consider the fact that all systems have boundaries. They can be permeable, semi-permeable or impermeable (rigid). And depending upon the state of the boundary, new information can flow freely or be blocked. And this fact is very important because systems tend towards balance or homeostasis, as I said earlier. Systems need to respond to unrestricted information flow, so they can adapt and change on the basis of this information.

Raxlen: What I see already in general systems terms is that for tick-borne disease we have a massive restriction on the flow of critical information that, if appropriately utilized, could change how we view the disease.

Bateson: I see a glimmer of light. I'm not ready to throw you to the feral cats just yet. I hope we have some time first for the principles of general systems theory. So, we need interacting units with communication linkages.

Raxlen: So, that means in this system we need to include spirochete bacteria, ticks, human and non-human warm-blooded mammalian hosts (mice, deer, chipmunks, moles) and vegetation ecosystems.

Bateson: And from what you have explained to me concerning the disagreements over the treatment of tick-borne disease, as it pertains to the flow and utilization or restriction of medical information, lets mix in physicians, insurance companies, state medical boards, Lyme group activists, government legislation at state and federal level, funding for further research…

Raxlen: I'm glad you mentioned those parts of the system because, if I look at the worldwide TBD problem, a recurrent question continues to repeat itself, with unfortunately a possibly malign answer. In the face of literally thousands of legitimate scientific articles published in the last 20 years that refute the inconsistent and inaccurate TBD testing paradigm which now exists, why is the narrow definition of Lyme symptoms, which excludes most patients who have been infected, still maintained? Why is the denial of the existence of 'chronic' Lyme, due to the obvious collusion between IDSA, CDC, insurance companies, research institutions receiving grant money and big pharma, still so pervasive? This kind of thinking keeps the system 'closed' and new vital information is choked at source. The field stagnates.

Bateson: You're right. From outside, the system resembles a scrambled hodgepodge. But let's organize it in such a way that we can capitalize on its insights.

Planet
Continent
Country
State or Region
City, town, neighborhood
Family / Extended family
Individual
Organ system
Multi-cellular
Cellular

If we explore tick-borne disease within this hierarchy of multiple-layered and interdependent systems, we can also start to identify the spots where we see problems that need to be repaired. It is my belief, that there are problems in every layer of the system when it comes to tick-borne disease.

Raxlen: I agree. And somehow, 'Lyme-literate physicians' must find a way to guide their patients to health despite all these bumps and snags along the way.

Bateson: Come to think of it, those microscopic bacterial friends of yours are definitely more fit to manage this situation then we are. Microbes were the first life forms on the planet. They have survived for billions of years without us. They were the supreme rulers of this uninhabited planet, colonizing every terrain possible from freezing arctic glaciers to sulphuric boiling undersea active volcanos. I suspect they will be here long after we're disappeared from Mother Earth. As to whether we blow ourselves up, or leave in a mass exodus in space ships for Mars, or some distant galaxy, will make no difference to them. They'll still be here on Earth, and always with us, or wherever we may be in the future. So long as humankind exists they will continue to be our symbiotic partners or our pathogenic enemies.

Raxlen: The adaptation of the borrellia spirochete is amazing. The tick ixodes scapularis abdomen is perfectly suited for the spirochete survival, which rises to inhabit the biting parts when the tick takes its blood meal. The spirochete also uses the tick's saliva, which is perfectly suited in its chemical composition, to allow the bacteria to enter the blood stream of the host unnoticed while the tick takes its blood meal.

Bateson: You have a worthy adversary, Bernard. I wish you luck in your medical endeavors. Just one final thought. A professor of cellular evolutionary biology, Lynn Margulis, theorized that our very cells are a symbiotic compromise between two early bacterial forms. Our DNA and the nucleus of every cell was once one type of bacteria, and the RNA of the mitochondria, our energy system, was another type of bacteria. They came together out of symbiotic necessity when the atmosphere developed its present concentration of then toxic oxygen, otherwise they would not have survived. I'm sure you are aware of this theory. It was originally scoffed at by the intellectual powers as fantasy, but now it has become substantiated by various molecular biology studies. She also hypothesized the origin of 'primitive nervous tissue' that responded to the environment in a purposeful way, for its own survival (light, temperature, food source, chemical composition) was derived from spirochete bacteria transmitting information via organized internal signals. Ultimately, she hypothesized that the primitive bacterial forms evolved into the nervous systems of all life forms and ultimately the architectural structure of our very brains. Like I said, Bernard, you have a worthy adversary who wears many disguises.

Chapter 12

The cadaver teaches – Empathy and emotional detachment

This next chapter, 'The cadaver teaches' will appear to be worlds apart from the abstract, rational systems theory 'metalogue' with Gregory Bateson, but they are connected by the fact that both, in their unique way, were significant influences on my personal development as a physician, intellectually and emotionally. Bateson gave me the understanding of systems thinking as it applied to complex problem solving in medicine. This in turn gave me a systems framework that connected linkages between independent units (i.e. family systems psychiatry and childhood aberrant behavior; double-bind communication and schizophrenic symptoms; depression and mold toxicity; general anxiety disorder and borreliosis etc).

What at first glance appeared to be unrelated data points (oak trees and acorns and white-footed mice populations, an increase or decrease in the incidence of TBD cases in any given year, predictable by noting acorn production, and how this in turn is related to the severity of climate change and deforestation), all these seemingly disconnected units could be linked into an interdependent system, where the whole was greater than the sum of its parts. A successful intervention into the system required knowledge of the system itself to avoid unforeseen negative consequences.

On the other hand, my encounter with a cadaver in the anatomy laboratory, which you are about to read, was a different experience for me. Not an enlightening intellectual experience like a Bateson lecture, but just the opposite; it was profoundly emotional. It opened my eyes to the stark fragility of 'human life'. It sensitized my ears to the 'silence'of the grave, and the silence was deafening. The cadaver spoke a special language – a wordless message that physicians don't want to hear. Some arm themselves by disengaging from their patients, or being coldly clinical. But there is no escape. The reality of the 'cadaver's truth' is Death. This was its silent lesson to me.

Medical school

Working as a young medical student, I remember the day I was exposed, for the first time, to a preserved formaldehyde-soaked human body. The original encounter was a shock. I have never forgotten it. It lies deep in a 'memory grave' but has zombie-like ramifications. I've realized over the course of years in practice, that this unholy part of my medical training had unconsciously affected my approach to patients, their health, sickness and death. Currently it extends to the diagnosis and treatment of tick-borne disease.

When the body was presented to me, I recoiled at the lifeless corpse laid out naked on the stainless steel, glistening, dissecting table, under the unforgiving glare of raw florescent lights. I was instantly nauseated. The grisly spectacle and the sickening, sweet, toxic smell of formaldehyde made me want to flee the scene. To protect myself, I realized at that very moment of this traumatic encounter, I had started to construct an emotional wall, shielding myself from the reality of the cadaver's truth. It is what the psychiatrist Dr Becker describes in his famous book *The Denial of Death,* the unconscious mechanisms we employ to deny the reality of the inevitable – namely, our own death.

I began on the very first day to treat the body as an object to be dissected. No humanity, no personal history, only an object to be examined and picked at with scalpel and tweezers. In order to survive emotionally, I was obligated to disassociate from the personhood of the cadaver and in so doing, distancing myself from the living patients that I was learning to treat.

Unfortunately, as medical students we can unconsciously carry this attitude into our daily lives as physicians, especially when we are confronted with an individual whose symptom presentation makes no sense – negative lab test results, negative diagnostic procedure results, failure of all applied technology to give coherent answers. If you can measure it, X-ray it, biopsy it, then the illness exists. To distance from the reality of the illness, and our helplessness derived from our own 'ignorance', we shift the blame to the patients themselves and 'behead' them. 'All in your head' is the common distancing phrase so often applied to tick-borne disease (TBD) patients.

TBD is an anathema to modern medicine because it follows no easy set pattern. The diagnosis is still, in the end, clinical. Laboratory testing, even in the best labs, is inconsistent with the clinical symptoms that the patient suffers. Treatment is individualized, dosing and the length of time medication needs to be administered are highly variable, ranging from three months to three years. Outcomes range from rapid, full functioning recovery to debilitating, wheelchair-bound, chronic, painful illness. It is little wonder that the unconscious wall of the physician is erected to deny the illness, avoiding its very reality.

How can a single unseen tick bite, with no known rash, or any proof of exposure, cause the patient such distress, physically, cognitively, emotionally? Faced with the 'strangeness' of this disease and its multiple combined systems involvement, and baffled by the persistence of the patient's condition after many attempts to treat the varying symptoms, there is a retreat to the dissecting table. We pick away at the disease, having to turn the patient into an inanimate object, denying the subjective experience of the TBD illness. Our ignorance then has to be the failure of the patient, certainly not the physician. My patients have so often told me that they have at times experienced a 'living death', with not a soul to turn to who understands their suffering. 'But you look so well,' people say, 'how can that be?'

The following essay was written more than 30 years ago for a presentation to a medical class reunion. It was never delivered because (for some reason that I don't remember) I was unable to attend the event. The original copy languished in my files all these years, and I came across it, quite by accident, in the process of writing this book. It illustrates how, as physicians, we learned 'unconsciously' the defense mechanisms of dissociation and projection and have applied them to Lyme disease and co-infections aka 'tick-borne disease'.

The cadaver teaches

In Leonardo's time, the 'dissection' was at best a 'crude and often revolting process'. Bodies for anatomical demonstrations came from the 'fresh carcass' of a recently executed criminal, quartered, mutilated often beyond recognition, in the last spasm of torture. The body, almost always 'male', was opened on a table by a barber in the winter, the cold for a brief time only slowing the bodily putrefaction. The barber demonstrated the 'foul viscera', while in a lectern above, the professor read aloud from the anatomical texts of the ancients. It didn't matter that the words read did not necessarily correspond to the evidence revealed by the flesh.

In fact, the evidence could be radically different. The point of the dissection was to confirm the words of the ancients, to uphold the traditional view. Investigation, to understand anatomical relevancy, was unheard of until Leonardo da Vinci. Cutting open the body was fraught with severe cultural disapproval and taboos. The idea that the body was the cosmos in miniature served to emphasize that with dissection came the possibility of interference in the perfect workings of God's creation. To cut open the cadaver was to violate blood both sacred and profane. Incision and dissection could in fact disturb the blood of Christ, or, worse, come in contact with the 'profanity' of menstrual blood. A too-curious quest for forbidden knowledge invited a deadly fate. To be a butcher, a barber or an executioner, or even a surgeon, was for the most part to be treated by society as an 'anathema' who risked divine retribution.

Picture, if you will, the following 'modern' medical anatomy class in contrast. A group of bright-eyed, now no longer pre-med, students are standing excitedly, congregated and eagerly awaiting entrance into our first anatomy class. We are in groups of four, going to be introduced to our five-day-a-week, 40-weeks-a-year, companion – our very own cadaver specimen. The air is tense with excitement. After all, isn't this what it's all about? Isn't this the reason for the insufferably long hours of study in the laws of physics and chemistry? Weren't we already being introduced to the perfume of formaldehyde, getting accustomed to it in the biology labs? Dogs, cats, fish, frogs, rabbits and mice were the unhappy victims of our dissecting scalpels. Wasn't the purpose of those unhappy hours to 'sensitize us' to the great adventure which lay in store for us? The interminable hours, the tests, the grades, the diagrams, the cookbooks and the dreaded finals were all behind us know. We had passed through the initiation of pre-meds and its untold demands, and were now waiting, almost not daring to breathe, for the anatomy room door to open. Now we were on the first leg of the journey to becoming doctors.

Without warning, the lab suddenly opened. The excited buzzing, which had a moment before electrified the air, was stilled. Four totally emotionless green lab-coated assistant demonstrators stood in front of the doorway and motioned us all without so much as a single word to follow them through the portals.

We entered, almost as if we had been hypnotized. The room was large, with hospital-painted-green brick walls. There were no windows, so air was being circulated by noisy overhead fans. The light was all artificial florescent illumination, which buzzed overhead in a muted hum. We were led to our anatomy tables in groups of four and told to sit on three-legged stools. One sense dominated the whole impressionistic kaleidoscope, and that was smell. The whole anatomy laboratory was permeated by the pungent odor of formaldehyde. It was a piercing presence, which felt to me as if I were breathing an alien atmosphere. The bodies lay before each of us, covered with a formaldehyde drenched oil-cloth sheet.

My senses were assaulted and my feelings ran the gamut of disgust through to morbid curiosity as to what lay under the sheet in front of me. I was also struck with another overwhelming wave of feeling, and that was a profound sense of melancholy and indescribable sadness.

And then, apparently out of nowhere, our anatomy professor materialized. He was a tall, lean Englishman, of mild, but very serious demeanor. He walked down the aisle between the dissecting tables and read from a list of names. He called each of us alphabetically and made a check mark with his pencil when we responded. Finally, he called my name, and it was as if he had summoned me to cross the river Styx. Like an automaton, I responded, 'Sir'.

When he had taken the roll, he stood in front of his blackboard. He picked up a pointer and without so much as minimal introduction or explanation, or reassurance about the strange and discordant situation we were facing for the first time, he simply stated his name and began his lecture as follows:

'Ladies and gentleman, my name is Dr Lister. I am your anatomy laboratory lecturer. These are my anatomy assistants. You would do well to consult them. They are here to help you with your dissection, should you need guidance. This is an opportunity for serious and important study. Anatomy has been the backbone of medicine for centuries. What you learn in this laboratory will be a vital link in all that you do in medicine in the future. This place is a place of dignity and a place for contemplation. This is not a rumpus room, nor a place of foolhardy antics. This is a place for hard and diligent work, painstakingly careful dissection, observation, note taking and weekly examinations. Not any of you here today in this class can graduate from medical school without having passed anatomy. This is not meant to intimidate you, it is simply the fact of the matter. Any questions?'

The room was deathly silent. No one spoke. Any questions? I have a thousand damn questions, but I don't know what they are. I just know that they are there. Stupid questions. Questions like, 'What the hell does this have to do with being a doctor and helping people? Why should it stink so much? Why aren't there any windows? No fresh air? Why does my whole medical career depend on anatomy only?'

I could imagine the reception I'd get if I asked those questions. 'Raxlen, this is an anatomy class, not a philosophy tutorial.' Still, the room remained deathly silent. Only the glaring overhead florescent lights hummed malevolently. Not one of us moved. No one asked a single question. All of the students were as intimidated as I was at this moment.

Dr Lister looked around the room, smiled a knowing smile, as if he had been through this boot camp exercise a thousand times, and then continued.

'Today we begin with the examination of the body superficially, and then move into the dissection of the hand. Understand that this specimen has been specifically prepared for dissection by my assistants. All veins and arteries have been injected with the special colored preservatives which will help you recognize them more readily. After you have thoroughly examined the body, both the outside and the inside, you will begin the dissection of the hand. Now, pay close attention, please observe and take notes.'

Lister then lectured in a dry monotone for another half hour or so. He drew from memory a perfect dissected hand in colored chalk, describing each set of relationships flawlessly. Bones, tendons, ligaments, vessels, nerves and finally muscles, were juxtaposed one on top of the other, weaving in and out to form a complex and intricate tangled complexity. When he finished, he put down his last piece of chalk and said, 'I expect all of you to be able to do the same by the time you are finished today.' He then walked the length of the room and turned to face us again.

'Ladies and gentleman, I hope your first day is enlightening. Now you may proceed.' And with that, he turned abruptly and strode out of the room. He disappeared for a full week.

And there we were, a classroom of ambivalent medical students, all eager to learn about the mysteries of the human body and to become caring physicians, but secretly unsure about whether or not we wanted to do it in this way. We all sat for a moment on our three-legged stools facing the formaldehyde covered body of our unknown human specimen. And then as if by a predetermined sign and joined by a common mind, we all pulled back our rubber sheets and stared at what lay in front of us.

I cannot say exactly, what every reaction of each of the medical students in the room was at that initial moment of confrontation. But I can remember the gasp that issued almost unconsciously from our throats. The sound was movingly eloquent in its uncensored inarticulateness. No experience of any kind had immunized us against the initial encounter with our cadaver. Death, and the preserved ruins of the human body, lay on our table, mocking each of us. And then, a storm of released energy broke across the room. A sudden, swift and unexpected cacophony of scrapping, shuffling, laughing, snickering and talking sounds filled the room and broke the tense silence. Students called across the room to others. Body parts were held up, cadaver arms were raised in greeting. Names were assigned to various bodies, like Mr Chips, Little Fred, Bubble Nose, Lucky Lady, Jane, Horace or Abysmal.

I remained silent and transfixed in front of my cadaver. It had once been a woman. Now, she was hag-like and strikingly toothless. Her mouth was just a dark hole, stuffed with formaldehyde-soaked cotton. Her face was other worldly, yet also somehow pathetically human. Her eyes were a greyish ochre opaque, and were directed at the ceiling at the bank of lights overhead. Lifeless eyes are particularly haunting and disquieting. They spoke of death with such finality. The skin was a parchment color and looked like a piece of leather that had been badly cured. The chest cavity and abdominal cavity had been flayed open to permit dissection. They too had been stuffed with a large wad of formaldehyde cotton to preserve the internal organs of the heart, liver, kidneys, bladder, uterus, lungs, etc. Her hips protruded forward, almost skeleton-like, with shrunken hollow flesh around the bony protuberances. Her pubis was prominent and matted with tufts of brackish thin hair. Grey-blue vulvular tissue was visible in the groin area. Her thighs and legs were shapeless pencils, flesh literally hanging from her bones.

So, this is what I have been waiting for, I thought to myself. This is it? I felt more like a macabre initiate than a medical student. I had to endure this in order to become a doctor? This was medicine in earnest. I wanted to flee immediately. I wanted to forget that I ever entered that sterile room of lifeless bodies. All around me was Death and the smell of formaldehyde. Death being picked apart scientifically and systematically, the better to understand life. Death defied by shiny sharp scalpels wielded by eager medical students. It took only 30 seconds for the sounds of my astonished classmates to subside. The novel assignment of dissecting a hand for the first time was undertaken with gusto.

I had no heart for it. I came to class, showed up to have my attendance taken, and watched my classmates do the work. I would observe morosely. I was involved in cadaver dissection only tangentially. I would obtain the lesson plan for the day, then leave as soon as possible and study the chapter in my anatomy book.

No surprise. I did very poorly in the subject. I barely passed, and only did because I memorized the textbook descriptions of body part relationships. I drew and redrew some of the key diagrams of major dissections. I kept a journal of sorts in which I entered intermittent impressions of those days. It provided me with a healing outlet for the despair I felt.

I reflected during those days: Who is this stranger? This unburied woman of no name? She who has passed through life's portals into the dark ignominious stillness of Death. She who lies so naked and grotesquely preserved. She, who we are dissecting with such meticulous resolve. From what mother love was she nourished? From whose family bosom did she emerge? What streets did she walk and through what doors did she enter and exit? How did she die? From what disease did she suffer? Was it just old age and being worn out by life? Who were her family? Her children? Her grandchildren? Who loved her?

I had thousands of questions. Thousands, upon thousands of them, none of which would be answered in the dissection lab.. Forty-five years and thousands of patients later, I still harbor thousands of questions about the lives I have engaged with as a senior physician. Lives that I have tried my very best to heal and make whole.

Some questions I have been able to answer. Other questions I have had to leave unanswered. Illness and Death were profound existential riddles posed to me by my silent cadaver. She proffered no answers to Life's mysterious energy, nor to its ultimate, often ignoble, ending. As a young physician in training I believed that surely medical science had all the answers. I was sure I would find solace in sophisticated medical knowledge to treat my patients correctly and shield them, albeit temporarily, from the cadaver's fate. At times I was, thankfully, successful. Other times I failed to stem the inexorable march of disease toward suffering and ultimately death.

Today I realize that we as 'homo sapiens', the most successful and dominant life form on the planet, may transcend 'disease' as we have known it over the entire history of mankind. I sense that in very short order, perhaps in less than 500 years, there may very well be a new species of intelligence which will dominate this planet – even beyond the planet's boundaries, even beyond our known solar system. Certain futurists believe that we are close to achieving a type of 'immortality'. Ageing, disease and death have been predicted to become an obsolete curiosity along with the cadaver.

Chapter 13

The Biography of a Germ The spirochete is psychoanalyzed

Arno Karlen PhD was a psychoanalyst in New York City who passed away some five or more years ago. He left behind writings on the history of medicine and biology. He had written essays on literature, general history, medicine and the behavioral sciences. In the year 2000 he published a little gem of a book about Lyme entitled *Biography of a Germ.*[62]

His book is written with the creativity and erudition of a first-class novelist weaving science, biography, history, fascinating facts and philosophical commentary into a spellbinding, uniquely original 6-inch by 8-inch, diminutive, 178-page book, divided into 25 miniature chapters. It is worth quoting a substantial part of his first chapter designated as 'A Very Small Life' because it elegantly outlines many themes found in this book:

> *To the naked eye, it is invisible, a nothing. Under the microscope it seems a silvery corkscrew undulating on a dark field. The form has simple elegance, like the whorl of a nautilus shell or the sweep of a dragonfly wing. But that simplicity is an illusion. Through the more powerful electron microscope you see not a featureless wiggle, but a shape-shifter – now a spiral, now a thread, now a rod or a sphere — with two walls, a dozen whiplike appendages and internal structures. And beyond any microscope's view, revealed only indirectly, by laboratory tests, lies a marvel of complexities. The surface bristles with molecules that sense and respond to the environment, and the interior churns like a chemical factory.*

Inside, more than a thousand genes flicker on and often changing sequences, to allow survival in places as different as a tick's gut, a dog's knee and a human brain.

It is the bacterium Borrelia burgdorferi, *by human standards a very small, brief flicker of life. Yet the boldest writer of science fiction could not invent a creature so ingenious, whose existence is entwined with that of so many other species. Although this microbe inhabits much of the earth and myriad hosts, it was not discovered until 1982, and then because it has ignited a new epidemic, Lyme disease.*

The illness so troubling to humans, is just a short, recent chapter in the germ's long history, and from its own perspective certainly not the most important one. Borrelia burgdorferi *has an ancient lineage, far older than ours, and despite all the vaccines and antibiotics we devise, it has a more promising future. It certainly preceded people on earth, and will doubtless survive us. For that very reason alone it deserves respectful biographers.*

Just as every person's life, seen close up, is compelling, so is every other creature's. Borrelia burgdorferi *is proof that if you want to see life afresh, and be struck with awe, you need only to take a 'germ's eye view' of the world.*

The book in fact does describe a 'little life', of a bacterium, in much the same way as any full-length biography of some significant personage. In that case the biographer would create the setting in which the selected person's 'life' would appear in its historical context; the biographer would elaborate on the setting, the time and place of the action. S/he would also relate the subject's ancestry, background, special friendships with others, struggles with adversaries, conquests and defeats, and the fame and fortune accrued to him or her.

Biographies of animals and insects, writes Dr Karlen, like biographies of people, also have a specific purpose. 'They illuminate the community of life, showing what makes species different and, more importantly, what unites them. They illustrate that by knowing any creature, great or small, one can better understand the living web in which it, and we, are threads. This is equally true of men and microbes. A corkscrew bacterium may lack the instant appeal of a kitten or a muskrat, but it, too, can evolve a sense of wonder and kinship. If, as Blake said, 'There is a miracle in a grain of sand,' there is much to amaze us in even the tiniest, least ingratiating creature. The life of *Borrelia burgdorferi* proves that life is never too small not to be compelling, or too short not to hold revelations.

But why Borrelia in particular?

Why would a psychoanalyst, of all people, write about Borrelia? Certainly the 'human condition' and human psychopathology are far more fruitful and interesting subjects for this type of professional. Dr Karlen goes on to explain why he chose this particular bacterium to write about:

> *Borrelia offers a biographer many traits rarely found together in one microorganism. First it illustrates a wide range of facts about bacterial life. It shows how species can coexist with a vast and varied biological community, an ability* Borrelia burgdorferi *(Bb) has in common with other widespread and adaptable organisms, such as us humans. Bb and its relatives reside in hundreds of species. from ticks to reptiles, birds and mammals. Despite this ubiquity, its relationships with its hosts are so specialized, that before Bb even enters a human, it must first reside in two or even three quite different creatures in a particular order. Thus, Bb's life presents a portrait in adaptation at a crowded ecological intersection. One can watch myriad species meet and change each other's lives.*

In the section written as a metalogue with Gregory Bateson, I outlined the importance of general systems theory and its application to TBD. Dr Karlen writes about the same 'general systems' subject matter, only alluding to it differently with different emphasis but obviously concerned about similar issues.

> *The Bb spirochete is affected by many changes in the environment, such as flora, climate change and changes wrought by human activity. More than most germs, Bb responds to hardships and opportunities created by deforestation, suburbs, global warming and cooling as well as people's shifting patterns of work and play. Although humans and Bb are two of the least similar organisms on earth, their lives and their fortunes are increasingly entwined —with us changing Bb's life at least as much as it changes ours.*

Of course, when one thinks of Bb, one thinks immediately of Lyme disease, sent over maliciously to mainland US some 40 years ago from Plum Island. A conspiracy theory implicates ex-Nazis gone rogue from the notorious, biological warfare centre. Nothing could be further from the truth. Bb and our ancestors have actually lived together for millions of years not bothering one another. Then in the last 10,000 years, give or take a few thousand, people started seriously messing around with their environment. They chopped down forests, cultivated the land, built villages and towns. Human animals for the first time began to seriously change their ecosystems and threatened the very survival of the germ. In fact, in some places it was almost wiped out! Borrelia genocide. However, the net effect over the last 10 millennia was that they both came closer together. A new balance evolved between the bacterium and its habitat.

Bb found new animal hosts, including humans, ready to offer them safe passage along with a delicious blood meal. Thus, Bb's altered ecosystem not only served its own needs, but was also a model for other microbes as well, which contacted human kind, their livestock and their pets. And it might have gone unnoticed if hadn't fired up the immune response so dramatically in its human host. And so, Lyme disease was born. And in less than 10 years after its discovery in Connecticut by a distraught mother, Polly Murray, it was found hiding everywhere worldwide. Now Lyme is rapidly increasing in frequency and rages over five continents – a not so well kept, age-old secret, hiding right before our very eyes for millennia. The undulating, silvery corkscrew has become a universal menace causing nothing less than a global pandemic. As Dr Karlen states:

> *Unlike many germs that enter people, Bb does not merely deliver a slap, fight a duel, and quit the field; it conducts a lingering campaign of biological warfare that can range over the entire body and last for years or decades. This encounter actually casts light on the nature of infection, host resistance, illness and well-being.*

There is an ironic twist to the Bb story writes Dr Karlen:

> *The irony is that it should have never have become a common human pathogen. Lyme disease is not epidemic because people raped the land, massacred other species [only themselves, my insert] or despoiled their ecosystems. Rather, it happened because people loved nature and became nostalgic for unspoiled settings; they tried to heal the land that they had unthinkingly exploited.*

To men like Gregory Bateson (see page 139), TBD is living proof that an ecosystem's complexity almost always exceeds our power to grasp it. And when we don't understand it, we set off a chain of mindless, bruising interventions which actually destroy the very system we are trying to heal.

But even as we start to understand it, once we choose to adopt Bateson's form of 'systems thinking' as an approach to the TBD pandemic, we can see issues that cause disruption of diagnosis and treatment at many levels of the system. Since TBD is a multi-microbial, multi-system disease entity, it affects not only the organ systems in the individual, but also other linked systems, which are arranged hierarchically. Information flows through the system in both directions, from complex to simple, and also from simple to complex.

A system is organized around units that interact with each other. These units taken together form an entity, in which the whole is greater than the sum of its parts. No unit can be understood in isolation. With TBD, we encounter 'negative feedback' at every level of the system. This starts as small as the invasion of the bacterium at cellular level, and the suppression of our immune systems, which in turn leads to negative testing and the dismissal of actual TBD patients. Or the failure of physicians to recognize symptoms arising from 'organ systems' that have become infected with Lyme and/or co-infection bacteria. Or the restricted definition of the illness by the CDC. Or the refusal to accept the existence of 'chronic', 'persistent', 'late stage' or 'advanced' Lyme disease by both the IDSA (Infectious Diseases Society of America) and CDC (the Centers for Disease Control and Prevention). This results in the failure of insurance companies to cover extended treatments and leaves patients stranded without resources.

At the medical organization level, the standard of care followed by most of the well-meaning physicians (i.e. three weeks of doxycycline) is unproven beyond the acute phase of the illness. The treatment fails to consider the sophisticated immune avoidance mechanisms of the bacterium, such as biofilm formation, round body or cystic formation, and cell wall deficient forms, all of which block antibiotic effectiveness (see page 109). In addition, the borrelia organism is immunosuppresive, since it can regulate B cells by altering their memory for recognizing foreign protein and increasing the inflammatory cytokine Il-6 as well as reducing IgG 1,2,3,4 (see page 247). A positive test through the two-tier system (ELISA and Western Blot – see page 65) is a necessary criterion imposed by the CDC and the IDSA for treatment. The incomplete science and exclusionary information upon which the IDSA guidelines rest, in 'systems' terms, are, in effect, 'negative feedback' information. This produces an error-driven outcome in the 'Lyme-system' as a whole. These supposed guidelines propagated throughout the medical community are nothing less than grave 'system errors' that continue to cripple the treatment of TBD. Negative feedback information is continually destabilizing the 'system' to the effect that clinically and scientifically correct information is suppressed or just ignored. Instead, 'system errors' are simply perpetuated to the detriment of treatment. This type of linear thinking also excludes from the 'system' the critical information pertaining to the complex problem of multiple co-infections.

We enter into a 'Lyme-system' where information errors are found at every level. The system becomes unstable, unbalanced and dangerous. The very patients it was supposed to help are crushed by its errors. The system becomes like a complex 'artificial intelligence' machine that has become hostile to its original program, like 'HAL', the malign computer in the film, *2001*. The end result is that it continues to produce more and more infected and untreated TBD patients. The unfortunate victims of the 'system' often find themselves on a slow, inexorable, slide into 'chronic unwellness', and a significantly diminished quality of life.

With the incredible polarization of TBD treatment here in the US and around the world, patients are caught in the middle. All physicians operate from unconscious premises since they perceive the world of medical illness through their unexamined biases. These principles of medicine have been taught in medical school, gleaned from the scientific studies that they have read (or not read) in leading medical journals, learned from the clinical experience of their colleagues at lectures and conferences, as well as from their direct clinical experience with their own patients. All of these factors coalesce to form their often-unexamined approach to treating a patient with TBD.

As in quantum physics theory, it has become axiomatic to view the 'observer' and the 'observed', or the 'experimenter' and the 'experiment' as a single continuum in which both parties are in a dynamic interaction with each other. It is not uncommon in medicine to have 'experimenter' bias affect the outcome and conclusions of an otherwise pristine scientific study. In the case of TBD, physician bias automatically limits the patient's narrative by reducing the amount of critical clinical information offered during the initial examination and in the ensuing visits. A distraught patient on her first appointment with me put it this way:

> *It was terrible. The specialist I saw spent no more than 10 minutes with me, tapped my reflexes, had me follow his finger, shone a light in my eyes and then said, 'It's definitely not Lyme. Frankly, I don't know what you have, but it's not too serious. Have you considered talking to a psychiatrist?' He then turned and walked out of the examining room and did not return. I was left sitting on the examining table in my ridiculous paper gown. I felt humiliated and confused, at the same time furious. I had the feeling that I was some sort of medical freak.*

The 'observer' (physician) directly affects what is being 'observed' (patient), while at the same time what is being 'observed' (the patient) in turn affects the medical information obtained by the 'observer' (physician).

It has been my experience that the physician's personality and character directly and dramatically influence the compliance and success of a patient's treatment.

So it is the responsibility of physicians to take care of the patients who enter their offices in search of a helping hand. We need to find a way to solve their problems rather than to dismiss them outright. This will involve more physicians looking for the 'commonalities' (page 16) as patients come through their office, but I think it will also require all physicians to take a more patient-centered approach to every case. I believe that the Physician-Activated Patient-Healing Response, as outlined above, will help every physician (regardless of where they stand on the Lyme debate) to better serve patients affected by TBD.

This problem is a big one. The CDC reports more than 300,000 cases of Lyme disease in the US every year, and this doesn't include the hundreds of thousands of cases outside the US, or those not diagnosed/misdiagnosed inside the US. It's time for us to come together, to recognize the scope of this problem and to start treating the whole patient, not just the flawed blood test result we see on their chart.

In the following section of this book, you will hear from a number of physicians, specialists and activists working with TBD around the world. Each country's fight against the epidemic is unique; the landscape is different in each culture. It is our hope that their chapters will help to guide patients around the world through the complex Lyme maze, and, as these authors work to raise awareness about the global scope of this problem, that they can also come together to form a unified front in the fight against this epidemic.

Part Four

A global epidemic

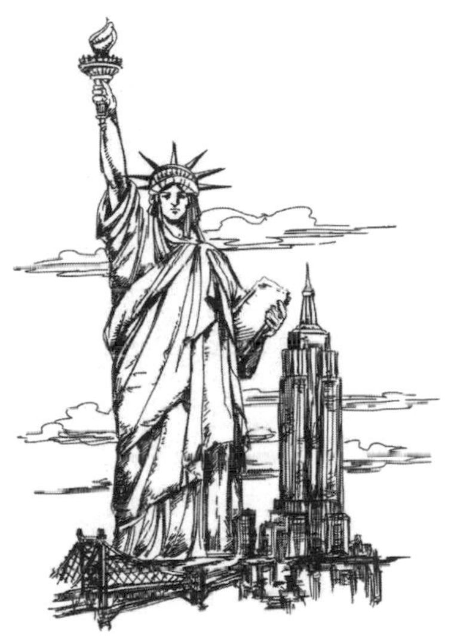

The following section features accounts from physicians and advocates around the world. It is our hope that these chapters will help to give a sense of the true scope of this epidemic and the effect that the Lyme maze has on patients and doctors in different locations. You will notice that the tick-borne experience globally is majorly influenced by the research, guidelines and practices of physicians in the United States. It is our responsibility in the US and elsewhere to change the paradigm, and to support the fight against tick-borne disease around the world.

We have included a brief biography of each author at the start of the book to shed light on their background and expertise.

Chapter 14

From New York, to the UK

Michael Cook

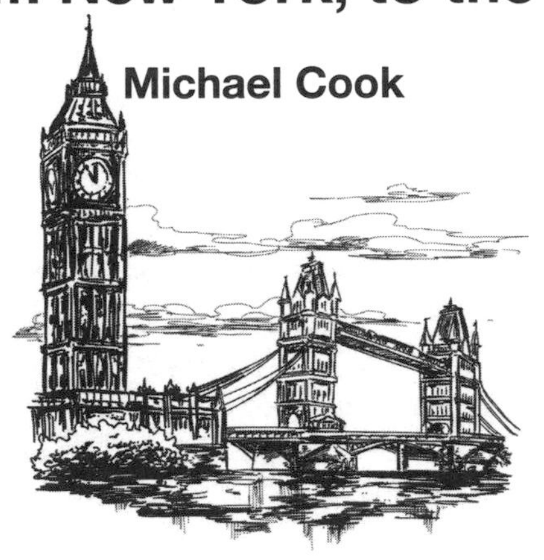

The history of Lyme disease in Europe precedes the naming of the condition. The first description of a Lyme-like rash in Europe was the report by Buchwald in 1883 of a 'diffuse skin atrophy' that had been present for 16 years in a 36-year-old patient.[63] The earliest known Borrelia infection in a human is from studies carried out on the 5300-year-old mummified body now named 'Ötzi' or the 'Iceman' discovered in the Alps between Austira and Italy. Based on samples extracted from bones and using 'next generation sequencing' and metagenomic analysis, DNA of *Borrelia burgdorferi* was identified.[64] The presence of Borrelia species in Europe was also determined from analysis of museum archive specimens. *B. garinii* was identified in ticks collected in Austria in 1884, and from British ticks collected between 1896 and 1994; *B. burgdorferi* family bacteria were found to have been continually present in the UK during that period.[65]

The first report of probable Lyme disease in the UK was in 1977, when Obasi, in a paper entitled 'Erythema chronicum migrans', described the case of a rash in a young boy.[66] This was followed in 1978 by a paper identifying six patients with erythema migrans (EM) rashes in East Anglia.[67] Possibly the first definitive report of Lyme disease in the UK was the 1986 paper describing a child admitted to hospital with fatigue, headache, stiff neck, photophobia and an expanding EM rash which subsided after five days. Serology testing identified Borrelia antibodies. The authors concluded with:

> *We cannot say whether our patient is an isolated curiosity, whether this particular illness has always been with us but unrecognized, or whether we may find ourselves with a new disease on our doorstep. We await the summer with interest…*

The title of the article, 'Lyme disease in a Hampshire child: clinical curiosity or start of an epidemic?'[68] with hindsight was highly 'prescient', and 30 years later the word epidemic is being used again.

Definition of Lyme

In the US, the name 'Lyme disease' was restricted to *Borrelia burgdorferi* infections transmitted by *Ixodes scapularis* ticks until 2017, when *Borrelia mayoni* was included. In Europe and the UK, other species of Borrelia and ticks have always been recognized as causing Lyme Borreliosis (LB). As of 2017, there were 51 named species of Borrelia with 21 classified in the LB group and evidence that nine are human pathogens. Two studies found the most common species present in the UK were *B. garinii* (61 per cent) and *B. valaisiana* (34 per cent), with *B. burgdorferi* and *B. afzelli* (3 per cent) and (2 per cent) respectively.[69, 70] *B. miyamotoi* has also been detected in the UK. *B. miyamotoi*, though classified in the 'relapsing fever' group of bacteria, causes Lyme disease symptoms, as demonstrated by Sato et al, where patients with a prior diagnosis of Lyme were actually infected with *B. miyamotoi*.[71] It does appear that some medical authorities restrict the definition of Lyme disease to specific Borrelia and Ixodes tick species, whereas a broader definition of Lyme borreliosis allows inclusion of all pathogenic species, and would more accurately reflect the true impact of tick-borne disease on health, common recommendations for avoidance and a unified guideline for diagnosis and treatment.

UK incidence and prevalence

In the UK, Lyme disease is not 'notifiable', although occupationally acquired disease should be reported to the UK Health and Safety Executive. Official statistics for England and Wales are based on data collected by Public Health England (PHE), which incorporated the former Health Protection Agency (HPA) in 2013, and by National Health (NHS) Scotland. The first official record reported 53 cases for the UK in 1996, and for England and Wales cases grew exponentially to 768 in 2006, with some ascribed to overseas travel. Recording criteria have changed a number of times and voluntary submissions from clinicians were excluded when 'enhanced surveillance' was introduced. From 2007 until 2012, incidence increased at a slower rate, to a level of 1040 cases by 2012. Reported cases then declined to 856 in 2014. Since 2014 the incidence has nearly doubled to 1579.

PHE and NHS Scotland suggest that incidence is two to five times higher than shown by official data, though the basis for these estimates is unclear. In addition to undiagnosed cases there are misdiagnosed cases, with evidence that Borrelia and other spirochetal bacterial infections contribute to diseases such as Alzheimer's. Also ME/CFS and other diseases of unknown etiology may be unrecognized Lyme borreliosis in some cases. The National Institute for Health and Care Excellence (NICE) stated in a report associated with the development of Lyme disease guidelines that there was a lack of epidemiological data in the UK and recommended research to determine the incidence.

The US Centers for Disease Control and Prevention reported in 2013 that three studies of clinician and insurance company data estimated that there were more than 300,000 diagnosed cases rather than their official figure of 30,000 – this is higher by a factor of 10 and still does not include undiagnosed and misdiagnosed cases.[72] The World Health Organization (WHO) stated that 85,000 cases were reported in 2010 for Europe;[73] however, a study by Müller et al indicated that in Germany alone there were over 200,000 cases in 2008 based on an estimate of 279 cases per 100,000 population.[74]

Misdiagnosis and undiagnosed cases result in an ever-increasing cohort of chronic illness of unknown proportions in the UK, Europe, USA and other regions

The medical system

The UK National Health Service (NHS) was founded in 1948 as a universal provider of medical care, free at point of delivery, funded by taxation. Over time, medical care based on insurance developed in parallel, funded by employers and private health services. Three major clinician groups diagnose and treat; general practitioners (GPs), accident and emergency doctors, and specialist consultants. In early 2017, the President of the Royal College of General Practitioners stated that doctors were 'ridiculously overworked' and that 'the average consultation length of 10 minutes in the UK – thought to be the shortest in the developed world – was crazy, and too short for complex health needs.[75] Accident and emergency clinic attendances have increased dramatically, and most of the Primary Care Trusts have large budget deficits. The King's Fund, an English health charity, stated in 2004:

> *As the UK population ages, growing numbers of patients will need help with managing complex, multiple conditions over sustained periods. This will pose significant challenges for the NHS, which will face both a large burden of ill health and vastly increased costs.*

This was in the introduction to a paper entitled: *Managing Chronic Disease: What Can We Learn from the US Experience?*[76]

These issues are now critical, with treatment choices being made based on cost/risk benefit analysis.

Diagnosis and testing

Lyme disease is difficult to diagnose due to the wide variety and variability of symptoms. With short consultations, high workloads and diverse illnesses, clinicians depend heavily on test results. Results from MRI scans, diabetes checks, UTI tests and blood counts are accepted as indicative of the presence or absence of a condition.

Lyme disease testing in the UK has predominantly been based on commercial test kits for the detection of antibodies, including Enzyme Linked Immunosorbant Assays (ELISA), Western Blot tests and occasional use of Polymerization Chain Reaction DNA testing. Tests are carried out by Primary Care Trust microbiology laboratories, the National Lyme Borreliosis Laboratory in Scotland and, up until 2012, by the Health Protection Agency (HPA) Lyme Reference Laboratory, Southampton. This laboratory was closed and its work moved in 2012 to the Rare and Imported Pathogen Laboratory at Porton Down. The accuracy of these tests, their sensitivity and specificity, have been extensively studied by independent researchers with results summarized in two reports.[77, 78] A study restricted to commercial test kits, including those used in the UK, demonstrated that sensitivity was near 60 per cent for samples proven to be from infected patients based on a definitive EM rash or prior positive serology. For early stage disease sensitivity was only 34 per cent.[79] Lyme borreliosis antibody tests have zero sensitivity immediately after infection and never achieve the accuracy of antibody testing for HIV for example. When used as defined in UK guidelines, with a screening test followed by a confirmatory Western Blot, the Lyme disease tests generate more than 500 times more false negative results than does HIV testing.[80, 81]

Additional problems with antibody tests that are not quantified include:

- Lack of test sensitivity data for species such as *B. valaisiana*, and others.
- Prior use of antibiotics or steroids which can prevent a detectable antibody response.
- Immune system variation (gender and age differences).

Clinicians are frequently uninformed regarding the limitations of Lyme disease testing and may even have been given questionable information. In 2010/11, the HPA stated on their website that:

> *Patients with late-stage disease are very seldom seronegative and there is a greater than 99% chance they will have a positive antibody response.*

However, the references cited did not support the claimed sensitivity.

In addition to the intrinsic lack of sensitivity of the tests used by the NHS, there are also problems specific to the testing laboratory. These can include:

- use of an 'inappropriate' test, such as one developed and certified for serum samples with cerebrospinal fluid without validation
- modification of the process parameters without validation
- modification of the manufacturer's instructions for interpreting results.

These issues can dramatically further reduce the accuracy of the tests and result in false negative results for thousands of patients.

Some patients with a negative UK serology test but strong suspicion of Lyme disease send samples overseas for testing. UK NICE guidelines say that tests should be carried out only at laboratories that are accredited by the United Kingdom

Accreditation Service (UKAS). UKAS is the body selected by the International Organisation for Standards (ISO) for certification to their standards for the United Kingdom. The PHE Rare and Imported Laboratory received accreditation to the ISO 15198 standard for Microbiology laboratories in mid 2018. ISO selects one certification body for each country, for example Deutsche Akkreditierungsstelle (DAkkS) is the ISO accrediting body in Germany. By defining that test results should be from a UKAS accredited laboratory by definition excludes laboratories from all other countries. However, the rules for defining positive samples with Western Blot tests are different in Germany, and using the same test kit, a sample considered negative in the UK could be positive in Germany. Commercial test kits are certified in the US by the Food and Drug Administration and in Europe with the CE mark of conformity. The CE mark is issued by Notified Bodies that are accredited by member states of the European Union. Neither the US nor European organization set a standard for test accuracy, only that the product meets the specification defined by the manufacturer. In the US, every microbiology laboratory must be approved by CLIA (Clinical Improvement Amendments Center). This requires that the laboratory meet defined standards for accuracy by correctly identifying positive, negative and equivocal samples provided by the agency. There are no independent organizations in the UK or Europe that have this function.

Development of UK guidelines

The evolution of diagnosis and treatment guidelines for the UK and many parts of Europe has been influenced by events in the US. One of the most important was a conference held by the Association of State and Territorial Public Health Laboratory Directors in Dearborn, Michigan in 1995.[82] Criteria for case definitions were defined by the Centers for Disease Control and Prevention (CDC) to ensure standardized reporting from the various states of the Union and avoidance of false positives. These were also adopted for clinical diagnosis. They required a history of EM rash and a positive two-tier test that used a preliminary ELISA screening test followed by a confirmatory Western Blot, as described earlier (pages 65, 183).

Although there had been earlier diagnostic and treatments guidelines published by Rahn et al and Burrascano,[83] the Infectious Diseases Society of America (IDSA) in 2000 published diagnosis and treatment guidelines.[84] An alternative set of guidelines was published by the International Lyme and Associated Diseases Society (ILADS) in 2004 which considered Lyme disease a complex infection that could be relapsing/ remitting and often refractory to antibiotic treatment, mirroring the work of Steere et al.[85]

Two influential groups formed during this time; the Ad Hoc International Lyme Group (AHILG), with 29 members primarily from US institutions and a representative from the UK Lyme Reference Laboratory,[86] and European Concerted Action on Lyme Borreliosis (EUCALB), formed with members from 14 countries. The release of updated US IDSA guidelines in 2006 was authored by 12 members of AHILG and two members of EUCALB.[87] In 2009, a German Lyme disease society complained that the use of these guidelines was extending beyond the US and the ability to treat patients was being adversely affected.[88] In 2010, the IDSA again updated their guidelines with no significant changes and similar recommendations were issued in a number of European countries, including for the UK by the British Infection Association (BIA). The BIA position paper indicated that serology testing using the two-tier test, with a screening ELISA followed by a confirmatory Western Blot, was the mainstay of diagnostic testing. A critique of the BIA guidelines was published by Lyme Disease Action, a UK charity registered in 1997, where they stated that limitations included unrealistic confidence in laboratory test sensitivity, bias in selecting supporting data and lack of evidence for the recommendations.[89]

Problems with guidelines

According to Shaneyfelt, problems have plagued guideline development and discussed the variable and opaque development methods and frequent conflicts of interest, both intellectual and financial. He commented that they often lack significant external review by stakeholders, and members of a clinical specialty are likely to recommend interventions for which their specialty serves a role.[90]

An independent study of IDSA infectious diseases guidelines determined that many were to a large extent dependent upon opinion, and that 50 per cent of the Lyme disease guidelines were based on opinion and not evidence.[91]

Examples of potential bias and conflicts of interest with Lyme disease guidelines include:

- Of the 29 member Ad Hoc International Group, 14 participated in writing the IDSA guidelines and many had interests in vaccines and/or Lyme disease test technology and patents.
- Many members of EUCALB represented microbiology laboratories and participated in the US and European guideline development, with some having patents related to testing and vaccines.
- All IDSA/EU guidelines require use of both of the two main competing serology test technologies, with a preliminary screening ELISA test followed by a Western Blot confirmatory test, with further testing for intrathecal production of antibodies to diagnose neuroborreliosis.
- A number of members of IDSA and AHILG have acted in disciplinary hearings. The manager of the Southampton Lyme Reference Laboratory declared a conflict of interest having acted as an expert witness[92] with more than 50 patient cases included in complaints to the General Medical Council against clinicians who had treated patients for Lyme disease.

- A number of AHILG personnel were retained as advisors to insurance companies.
- An investigation of the IDSA Lyme disease guideline authors by the Attorney General of Connecticut resulted in a 2010 report that stated: 'my office uncovered credible evidence of undisclosed conflicts of interest and other significant flaws in the process that produced the guidelines.' Currently (February 2019) there is no active IDSA guideline with the 2010 version placed in the society archive.

In 2017, after representations to the government by the Caudwell Lyme charity, the Department of Health assigned development of UK guidelines to the National Institute of Health and Care Excellence (NICE).[93, 94] The committee was led by Professor Saul Faust, a Pediatric Immunology & Infectious diseases consultant, with 14 other member including clinicians and members of the public.[95] There were members that specialized in infectious diseases, though no members of the committee were published authors on Lyme disease recorded in PubMed. Extensive consultations with stakeholder groups and literature searches identified over 2400 studies which were used to generate a reports of more than 1800 pages. The completed guideline was published in April 2018.[96] A follow-up report indicated that of the 15 recommendations 10 (66.7 per cent) were based only on the experience and opinion of the Guideline Committee members, three (20 per cent) were based on experience and opinion including very low evidence, one (6.7 per cent) recommendation was based on low quality evidence and one (6.7 per cent) defined as moderate to very low.[97]

Some important statements include:

The erythema migrans rash 'increases in size'. This often-quoted comment may have resulted in clinicians recognizing the rash, which is definitive for Lyme disease, but not treating unless there was evidence of an increase in size. The rash does expand but not indefinitely and may have reached maximum size when seen by the clinician. An EM rash of any size is clinically diagnostic though the CDC and other require a rash greater than 10cm for surveillance reporting. In the diagnosis section it states that Lyme disease is an 'uncommon' cause of symptoms such as fatigue, migratory joint or muscle aches, headache or cognitive impairment. However, as previously mentioned NICE in their reports stated: 'there was a lack of robust epidemiological data on Lyme disease for the UK population', and that 'research was needed'. Hence the statement that the disease is uncommon is not founded on robust statistical evidence which the committee decided did not exist.

The guidelines recommend that a clinician should ask if the patient's activities might have exposed them to ticks and if they had travelled to areas where Lyme disease is known to be highly prevalent. However, the clinician would not know whether the patient is educated in the epidemiology of Lyme disease and also the relevance of the question must be questioned since the committee state in Section 1.1.1 of the guideline that:

- 'Ticks are mainly found in grassy and wooded areas, including urban gardens and parks';
- 'Infected ticks are found throughout the UK and Ireland, and although some area appear to have a higher prevalence of infected ticks, prevalence data are incomplete.'

Hence, it is not necessary to travel to a 'hot spot'; the patient may have infected ticks in their own garden or where they walk the dog each day.

The committee stated: 'evidence on the effectiveness of antimicrobial treatment regimens used in different presentations of Lyme diseases is of poor quality, outdated and often based on small studies.' However, the guidelines give very precise instructions for antibiotic types, dosage and duration and limits for use by GPs. There is evidence that a number of conditions respond in time to long-term treatment with antibiotics. In 2010 the World Health Organization (WHO) increased recommended treatment time from 2 months to 6 months for tuberculosis to reduce treatment failures,[98] and they released guidelines for leprosy in 2018 with a recommendation for a three-drug treatment protocol including Rifampin and Dapsone of 12 months duration for multibacillary leprosy.[99]

Patient experience of the medical system

There are many clinicians diagnosing and treating Lyme disease with varying degrees of success. However, there is little published research on the patient experience. Major sources of information are national and local news services, with an increasing number covering personal stories and interviews with celebrities and the general public. These frequently share a common theme of severe, life-changing illness with an inability to function in careers, education and normal daily routines. They document multiple interfaces with a wide variety of clinicians, receiving many different diagnoses, especially with illnesses that have vague or unknown causes, such as ME/CFS, anxiety and depression. The reports sometimes include that by privately funding diagnosis and treatment, the patient's symptoms have resolved or they have gained significant relief from the illness. These anecdotal reports make the headlines, and when patients have exhausted all possibilities within the NHS, they turn to alternatives, including private treatment. Some patients sell their homes and use the equity to fund their treatment; others use savings or inheritances, and occasionally crowd-sourcing campaigns raise the funds needed for treatment. These are desperate measures, clearly undertaken by desperate people.

Internet websites, blogs and social media have dramatically changed the way information is shared and these resources are widely used by Lyme disease charities, support groups and patients. Commonly featured are reports of patient-clinician encounters that disturb and are sometimes devastating for patients. Anecdotal reports of statements from clinicians include:

- There is no Lyme in this area (stated in a highly endemic area).
- Your tests are not positive enough.
- It's stress; here are some antidepressants.
- There's nothing wrong with you; you just think you have Lyme disease.
- You have too many symptoms for an infection; it is all in your head.

And from patients include:
- My clinician was told to stop treating me after talking with the Lyme specialist because the test was negative.
- All the consultants I saw were dismissive and rude.
- I was treated as if I was faking it.

In order to obtain evidence of patient experiences and the views of clinicians in the UK, the Department of Health commissioned a study by the EPPI Centre at University College London (part of London University). This group, established in 1993, informs policy makers using systematic reviews. Specialist teams from the EPPI Centre at University College London, the University of York, and the School of Hygiene and Tropical Medicine were used to study issues related to knowledge in four areas:
- Incidence of Lyme.
- Experiences of Lyme diagnosis.
- Experiences of Lyme treatment.
- Prevention of Lyme.

Each study followed a standard evidence gathering and assessment methodology. Publication of the reports was in December 2017 with extensive information from each group. There were many important conclusions including:
- The analysis of studies on the incidence of Lyme disease showed they were mainly from the US with others from Europe, none were from the UK and quality assessment scores ranged from zero to 7 out of a possible score of 40.

- Of over 1000 published papers related to populations affected by Lyme disease there were very few that focused on potentially at-risk groups with only 10 on Hikers / Outdoor pursuits, two on pet owners and two on older people. Only 5 per cent of papers were from the UK.
- Very few papers covered the clinical / symptom diagnosis, with little research on risk factors and costs.
- Research was urgently needed for implementation of effective treatment.
- Studies indicated that clinicians found it challenging to diagnose Lyme disease accurately, and some called for a more accurate test. Also patients experienced difficult journeys to obtain diagnosis and treatment, with ambivalence or skepticism from clinicians.
- There were negative consequences, both emotional and financial.
- Patients and clinicians agree that clinicians lack sufficient knowledge of the disease and that quantitative research is needed.

In addition to the evidence-based studies in 2017 the EPPI group carried out face-to-face meetings with eight patient advocacy groups.[100] Every advocacy group reported that patients believed they were 'denied' a diagnosis, with clinicians:

- stating 'Chronic Lyme disease does not exist.'
- stating 'I don't deal with Lyme disease.'
- 'laughing at me when given my private test results.'

A strongly expressed view was that diagnosis was delayed because the full spectrum of symptoms was not recognized: cardiologists viewed the heart, dermatologists saw only a rash, and patients were 'pushed from pillar to post'. Initial and frequently multiple cases of misdiagnosis was given as a cause of delay in getting treatment that targeted Lyme disease.

An internet-based self-selected patient survey carried out in 2014 provided inputs to an EPPI study.[101] It indicated that misdiagnosis was common, with patients reporting the following diagnoses:

- Chronic fatigue syndrome 48 per cent
- Viral infection / post viral syndrome 34 per cent
- Anxiety / stress 32 per cent
- Depression / psychiatric illness 31 per cent
- No diagnosis given 30 per cent
- Fibromyalgia 21 per cent
- Multiple sclerosis 4 per cent
- Other 37 per cent.

Other diagnoses included: arthritis, Bell's palsy, bipolar disorder, contact allergy skin rash, Guillian Barre and many more. The average number of times they were misdiagnosed was three; however, there are reports of many more visits to clinicians over a period of years or decades before a diagnosis of LB and treatment.

These findings support the longstanding anecdotal reports that have circulated by word of mouth and on social media platforms for many years.

The most important factor that governs the patient experience of the medical system is the interface with clinicians. Few clinicians will have received information specific to Lyme disease at medical school, and will depend heavily on the influence of respected journals, medical associations and the Department of Health. Examples of the positions expressed include an article in the *Lancet* entitled: 'Antiscience and ethical concerns associated with advocacy of Lyme disease'.[102] This unfairly conflates the groups that deny the viral cause of HIV with Lyme patients and their support groups. The article also claims that advocates have created pseudoscientific research and publications to subvert evidence-based medicine. This is simply an attack on all research that does not fit their view, when in fact it has been carried out at respected institutions and published in peer-reviewed journals. There is a potential conflict of interest in that a number of journals are house organs of the IDSA, and 12 members of the Ad Hoc International Lyme Group and EUCALB are on the editorial boards of many journals, with two members being editors of more than 20 journals each.

Patient-advocate position

- Lyme disease occurs on almost every continent
- Borrelia has antibiotic-tolerant forms
- A short course of antibiotics may not be effective
- Lyme disease can be a chronic disease and can respond to longer courses of antibiotics.

Ad Hoc International Lyme Group position

- Lyme disease is limited geographically
- Lyme disease has no antibiotic-tolerant forms
- The disease is responsive to antibiotics
- Persistent symptoms are due to tissue damage or a post-treatment syndrome.

Occupational exposure

Epidemiological studies indicate that high levels of borrelial infections are associated with employment, with seropositive blood samples from farmers, forestry and park workers, military personnel and veterinarians. Sample are typically in the range 15-30 per cent seropositive though can be over 40 per cent. Examples from 40 papers published on seroprevalence infection rates in various populations are:

- Austria 1988 Military recruits 20 per cent,[103]
- England 1989 Foresters 25 per cent and Farmers 14 per cent,[104]
- France 1993 Farmers 39 per cent,[105]
- Italy 1993 Rangers and Foresters 19 per cent,[106]
- Netherlands 1991 Foresters 20 per cent.[107]

These reports usually defined the groups as asymptomatic or healthy. One study of orienteers over a period of seven years showed that 4.9 per cent of the seropositive cases developed clinical Lyme disease with an annual rate of 0.8 per cent, which represents an annual LB incidence of 800 cases per 100,000;[108] 26 per cent seroprevalence of IgG anti-*Borrelia burgdorferi* antibodies was observed among 950 orienteers and the incidence of new clinical infections was 0.8 per cent. In 1993, a total of 305 seropositive orienteers were re-examined. During that time, 15 cases (4.9 per cent) Rath et al, in a study with follow up after six months, commented that: 'clinical signs were rare', however, in the discussion section they stated: 'the incidence of clinically manifest illness within the observation window of six months seems low (about 2 per cent)'. If this 2 per cent is extrapolated to one year it represents a 4 per cent incidence of disease which is 4000 cases per 100,000 population. A study of Dutch forestry workers by Kuiper et al, with a one-year follow-up, found that five of 95 (5.3 per cent) workers converted from negative to positive in antibody tests and two (2.1 per cent) workers had clinical symptoms of Lyme borreliosis. This represents a disease incidence of 2100 cases/100,000, and an infection incidence of 5300 cases per 100,000. This again is an extraordinarily high rate and conversion from seropositive to symptomatic clinical Lyme borreliosis cannot be considered rare. Whilst there are no similar studies reported for the UK there is no reason to doubt that similar statistics prevail.

Although the disease is notifiable in the UK if occupationally acquired, the financial liability of large numbers of people medically unfit to work will be very high. Since Borrelia infections occur at any age and frequently in the young and middle aged the cost of funding disability payments for 30, 40 or more years would be extraordinarily high.

Summary

It is clear that, since the initial reports and studies on Lyme disease, there has been a distinct change in the Lyme story. The very first reports indicated a disease of epidemic proportions with a prevalence of over 400 cases per 100,000 population and 10,000 cases per 100,000 in children. In many cases it was unresponsive to antibiotics, and symptoms included 'profound' fatigue.[109] Later it was defined as 'rare' and successfully treated with a 'short course of antibiotics'. Meanwhile, great efforts were made to develop vaccines, which after over 30 years have still not been effective, with a major vaccine manufacturer abandoning development in 2012/13.

Poor test sensitivity and lack of recognition of symptoms has resulted in late diagnosis and lost opportunities to treat the disease soon after infection. At that stage, before the bacteria are widely disseminated, short courses of low-cost oral antibiotics are generally effective. In the later stages, where major organs including the brain and heart are affected and with neurological complications, treatment guidelines suggest intravenous antibiotics with the associated risks and costs, and with high levels of treatment failure.

For whatever reasons, over the last 30 years or so the disease has been misrepresented in incidence, severity and treatability. Reasons may relate to vaccine and test development, patent royalties, cost/risk analysis and/or burden shifting from healthcare to disability budgets. The consequence is that there is a group of people of unknown but ever-growing size, left suffering from a debilitating, life-changing and sometimes life-ending condition. This group is generating high but unknown costs to medical systems and disability benefit programs. Additionally, it is a major burden not only in terms of ill health of the patient, but also for their carers, family members and friends.

Chapter 15

Lyme disease in Ireland

Dr John Lambert

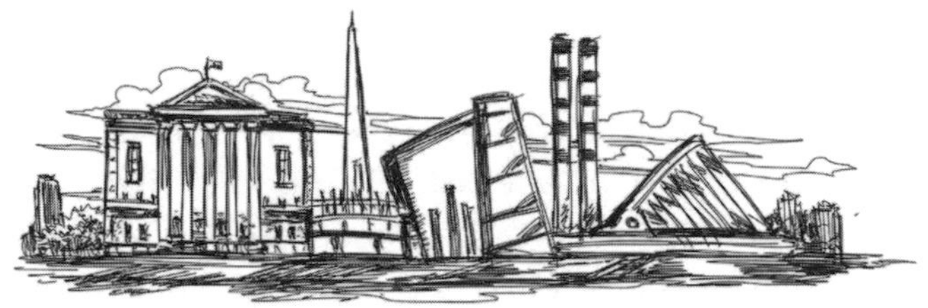

In Ireland, Lyme is a disease with significant political contention surrounding its diagnosis and treatment. It is an area that generates much disagreement between patients and doctors, and within the medical profession itself.

Treatment guidelines

The most widely accepted guidelines for the clinical management of Lyme borreliosis are those of the Infectious Diseases Society of America (IDSA): *Clinical Assessment, Treatment, and Prevention of Lyme Disease, Human Granulocytic Anaplasmosis, and Babesiosis: Clinical Practice Guidelines*.[110] These guidelines were endorsed in a consensus statement issued in 2012 by the Scientific Advisory Committee of the Health Protection Surveillance Centre,[111] the Infectious Diseases Society of Ireland, the Irish Society of Clinical Microbiologists, the Irish Institute of Clinical Neuroscience and the Irish College of General Practitioners. This statement says that 'these guidelines represent the best and most effective synthesis of the available evidence on the treatment of Lyme disease'. Most infectious disease clinicians in Ireland are members of the IDSA in the US, as many current consultants spent training years in the US learning their areas of expertise, and tend to support the IDSA documents. Most are not aware that the IDSA guidelines for Lyme are 'under review', and stick to the mantra that patients can receive only 'one month of doxycycline' for Lyme, describe any symptoms following that one month of treatment as 'post-Lyme'(implying resolved infection rather than ongoing infection) and decline to believe there is ongoing infection; they also do not generally consider the possibility of 'co-infections'. They debate the issue of 'chronic Lyme', stating it does not exist, and also are critical of alternative guidelines, including the ILADS (International Lyme and Associated Diseases Society) and German (see below) guidelines. This is despite there being many scientific publications that show Borrelia persists for long periods of time with and without treatment.

Thus, alternative guidelines for the treatment of Lyme and tick-borne disease (TBD), such as those produced by ILADS or the German Borreliosis Society, have seen little mainstream recognition or support in Ireland. I (Dr John Lambert) am an exception to this 'mainstream'. I had significant experience in Lyme disease and co-infections in my work in the US prior to returning to the UK in 2000, and I have been working as an infectious disease clinician and researcher in Dublin since 2005. I have been establishing a platform for research and clinical care for Lyme patients, where others would not see them, or where others dismissed their complaints as psychosomatic or worse. My practice provides a multi-faceted approach to treatment, utilizing the ILADS guidelines, and also building on antibiotics with natural supplements, immune modulators, natural anti-inflammatories and 'complementary therapies', all of which are necessary for treating TBD as all of these issues – infection, inflammation and autoimmunity – need to be addressed to cure these infections.

Chapter 15

Diagnosis

In Ireland, early Lyme disease is primarily a clinical diagnosis, made by taking a medical history and undertaking a physical examination of the person. There are very few clinicians with experience of diagnosing Lyme, and little awareness that the disease exists and is endemic in Ireland, as there are incomplete statistics and epidemiological studies. Sadly, many general practitioners (GPs) tell their patients that there is 'no Lyme in Ireland', as there are no statistics relating to its prevalence. And there is no training at GP level to change that opinion. Furthermore, when patients present with the classic EM (erythema migrans) rash, even when the patient identifies the rash following a tick bite, clinicians often come up with an alternative diagnosis, such as 'ring worm' or 'cellulitis'. However, the guidelines say that if the characteristic EM rash is observed, antibiotic treatment should be initiated without the need for further follow-up confirmatory testing. Very often, treatment is not given as doctors wait for the antibody test, and decline to give patients treatment in the absence of a positive result. In the absence of a visible rash, two-step laboratory testing (see page 65) is conducted, in accordance with IDSA guidelines. Laboratory tests are needed to confirm a diagnosis of later stage infection. The 'two-tier' test is fraught with all of the problems that have been previously identified, but the Irish guidelines state that their antibody screening tests are close to 100 per cent accurate. Other scientific studies show less than 50 per cent sensitivity of this 'standard' test. Why? There appear to be other strains of Borrelia that exist in Ireland (see below) that are not being picked up by the 'standard' test that was developed for the original American isolate.

Data regarding the prevalence of Lyme in Ireland are limited, as I have said. Only Lyme neuroborreliosis, a more severe neurological manifestation of Lyme disease, is monitored as a notifiable disease. So only a few dozen cases are reported to the government annually, and these are the numbers used to assess the 'burden of disease'. Without any regulatory onus on doctors to report cases, it is difficult to ascertain how widespread Lyme is. Notification allows identification in a more systemic way and helps in following trends in the disease over time. Accurate monitoring of disease in humans, animals and tick vectors will be a necessary step in Ireland as a first step to give accurate statistics on disease burden.

Lyme disease is a diagnosis that is often overlooked by clinicians. Despite the considerable evidence that a significant proportion of the Lyme cases seen in Ireland have been exposed locally, individuals displaying symptoms are much more likely to be tested for Lyme (for example, even if they give a history of recent travel to the Northeastern US and were bitten or had a 'flu like illness) . Even in Kerry, Connemara and Donegal, areas of Ireland well known for ticks that carry Lyme, Lyme-literate clinicians are rare, and many GPs are dismissive of patients who raise the issue of Lyme.

The Irish travel throughout the world and often are exposed to many pathogens, including tick-borne varieties, but a recent audit in my clinic has identified likely exposures within Ireland from Donegal, the Wicklow mountains, Kerry, Sligo, Waterford and Connemara. Outside of Ireland, patients travelling in the UK are evaluated with a history of likely exposure in northern Scotland and the Border counties, Northern Ireland (County Down) and Northern Wales. The Irish also frequently travel to North America (US and Canada, with Vancouver as a frequent location), Europe (especially France and Germany), Eastern Europe (Slovenia, Poland, the Baltics), and the Canary Islands, where a number of different varieties of Borrelia and co-infections have been identified in the tick populations.[112]

In addition, Ireland has a large Eastern European population, who often spend their summers in the Balkan states and Poland, and return unwell with 'flu-like' illnesses. They may or may not have a rash. Many Irish practitioners do not include Lyme as part of the differential diagnosis when evaluating such patients.

There is evidence that Lyme disease is moving northwards as temperatures rise due to climate change, facilitating a rise in the numbers of mammal and bird hosts for the ticks. This means that diagnoses of Lyme must be considered in areas outside those traditionally considered endemic.[113]

People at highest risk of the disease are those walking through woodland and other country areas. In Ireland, farmers and outdoor workers are disproportionately infected and affected. One needs to consider the diagnosis in travellers returning from camping and hiking holidays from EU countries where Borrelia is more common, as well as those returning from the Eastern US and other parts of North America. The Irish frequently travel to these regions, as well as acquiring these infections at home.

As I have said, a major issue surrounding the diagnosis of Lyme in Ireland is that the strains of Borrelia most often found here and in the rest of Europe (*Borrelia afzelii* and *Borrelia garinii*) are distinct from those common in North America (mainly *Borrelia burgdorferi*). As a result, it is possible that the testing standard currently used in Ireland is missing patients infected by strains of Borrelia predominant in Europe. In fact, the Irish laboratories specifically state that their tests are close to 100 per cent accurate in diagnosing Borrelia (synonymous with 'Lyme' as used here), but on further questioning they do not clarify that their test only identifies *B. burgdorferi* and does not take advantage of the data throughout other European countries that have identified the other strains – *B. afzelii* and *B. garinii* – as the predominant species in those regionally infected.[114] As practitioners in Ireland are not 'Lyme literate', they depend on the interpretation of the reporting laboratories in Ireland, and often do not put the history, clinical picture and laboratory testing together to make an appropriate diagnosis, leaving the patient destined for a long course of chronic undiagnosed disease.

A further potential pitfall when it comes to current diagnostic standards is the possibility of a patient with undiagnosed Lyme who may not produce the necessary antibody response due to a compromised immune system. The testing reports do state that it is a 'clinical diagnosis' but as most clinicians do not know how to recognize the EM rash, and up to 50 per cent of patients do not have the classic rash anyway (although the Irish guidelines say 80 per cent will have it[115]), there are lots of opportunities to miss a Lyme diagnosis in Ireland. Many believe the EU strains are less likely to give a classic EM rash than the American strains, but most of the sources of medical information used by the Irish system are US-centric.

As we cannot culture Borrelia with current technologies, we have turned to newer immunological laboratory diagnostic tests, such as the 'ELISpot LTT' (see page 243) and CD57+ tests currently being offered to people in Ireland by private German laboratories; these show promise as a reliable alternative to the currently accepted two-tier antibody testing. These are 'ELISpot assays', which are immunological assays that give indirect evidence of exposure to the infection as measured by a gamma interferon release measurement following exposure to the tested antigen/suspected infection; this same technology is being used in all Irish hospitals to assist in the diagnosis of latent or active tuberculosis (the 'TB quantiferon assay'). When Irish specialists are given the Borrelia ELISpot LTT assays by patients who have gone to Germany as they are unhappy with the current standard of care being given in Ireland, the comments from these clinicians will be that 'the German labs are not accredited, and that all patients have positive German ELISpot results', and that the tests are of no value. The reason for these unprofessional and scientifically unfounded comments is not clear. While the ELISpot assays to Borrelia and other tick-borne bacteria are new technology, many patients in Ireland have had a tick bite, had a negative standard screening assay done, been told they do not have Lyme based on the standard Irish Lyme test (which misses the diagnosis in many situations), and then sought alternative testing. And when the testing done in these private laboratories has given a positive result, and even when these patients have got better on treatment given by Lyme-literate physicians, traditional doctors in Ireland will still denigrate the tests and question the therapies given. These are often patients who have been sick for years, having been seen by many medical specialists, none of whom has been able to diagnose the patient's problem or get the patient better with any of their 'specialty' treatments, whether they are neurologists, rheumatologists or other consultant specialists. Patients are told these laboratories are 'not accredited' but indeed all of these EU laboratories have internationally recognized accreditation, the same as Irish laboratories. However, the 'daisy chain' of whispers and misinformation is spread from consultant to GP to patient, and patients are denied treatment. Occupational health doctors deny patients in Ireland work and insurance benefits as they state in their reports the laboratories are not accredited. Medicine by wrongful whispers should be challenged by patients as they have rights to care, and the medical and legal system should protect them and support them.

Moving forward

As we move forward, it will be important to teach clinicians that following a tick bite, or a suspected tick bite, people should not be tested just for Lyme (Borrelia). Co-infections and other diseases that display similar symptoms should also be considered. Many doctors are not aware of other tick-borne infections – such as Anaplasma (page 58), Babesia (page 52) and Rickettsia (page 54). Other infections acquired by the respiratory route (e.g. Chlamydia pneumonia, Mycoplasma pneumonia) can cause chronic systemic disease and be a contributing factor in the clinical presentations of 'Lyme-like' infections. For many patients suffering from Lyme-like conditions, there may not be one unifying diagnosis, but multiple pathogens contributing to their condition. While Lyme-literate physicians understand this, 'traditional' medical practitioners question the existence of a pathogen causing 'chronic Lyme-like conditions' that can be cured with antibiotics.

The term 'post-treatment Lyme disease syndrome' has been used by IDSA and their followers to de-emphasise the role of ongoing infection by Borrelia and other co-infections in patients with chronic symptoms. There are many animal and human studies that show persistent chronic infection following acute infection; these are often ignored or just not quoted. This condition is untreated infection, or partially treated infection. To give patients a diagnosis of 'post treatment' when they are still infected, and indeed respond and get cured with longer courses of antibiotics, is an experiment that many liken to a human rights violation. Other patients with spirochetal infections have been denied treatment, the notorious 'Tuskegee Study of Untreated Syphilis in the Negro Male' (1932 to 1972) being the landmark case. Patient groups in Ireland and politicians have taken the lead in advocacy as the government and most consultants and GPs have let their patients down.

Given that current diagnostic techniques are imperfect, and many patients with antibiotic-treatable infections are being missed, we have established a specialist service in Ireland that has been evaluating patients with Lyme-like clinical conditions where a clear diagnosis has not been established by standard testing algorithms.

In our private infectious disease clinic in Dublin, an audit was conducted of 100 patients presenting with 'Lyme-like' symptoms. The majority of these patients had had previous diagnoses of 'chronic fatigue syndrome' or 'fibromyalgia' without an identified explanation for their symptoms.

These patients were carefully selected for review based on their history. Most of them had previously been healthy but within the recent past had had a sudden unexplained onset of illness followed by continuing ill health. These patients had then run the gamut of undiagnosed illness for many months or even years, going to many specialists and being given multiple diagnoses, none of which had really fitted their clinical symptoms. Results from this audit indicated a significant prevalence of infections such as anaplasmosis and Chlamydia pneumonia, among others. In this group of patients who were negative for Lyme by standard antibody testing, ELISpot assays were performed against Borrelia antigens, and they tested positive for Lyme by this method.

And following a diagnosis of chronic Lyme/co-infection, almost 70 per cent of patients responded to combination longer-term antibiotics. Based on this audit, and other similar studies in the literature, patients with a wide variety of rheumatological and neurological diseases have been found to have an infectious explanation for their condition previously diagnosed as some other condition (ME, CFS, FM), and indeed such patients responded significantly, or had total resolution of their disease, with individually chosen combinations of antibiotics and supplements, administered in combination for 'longer' periods of time than current IDSA recommendations allow. These patients had previously been diagnosed with 'atypical' syndromes.

As we currently have no 'recognised' antigen-specific tests to make a diagnosis of these conditions, we must use clinical judgment. We treat longer for other infections if patients show a response to treatment and do not restrict antibiotic treatment for cellulitis or bone infections; if patients get better with longer courses of treatment for these conditions, we should be allowed to use clinical judgment, just as for other infectious diseases conditions,

Building awareness

Continued efforts have been made by patient advocates to elevate the profile of Lyme and tick-borne disease in Ireland. Tick Talk Ireland, Ireland's first Lyme disease support group, was set up in 2009 with the goal of encouraging awareness, prevention and treatment of Lyme disease in Ireland. It continues to conduct numerous awareness rallies, talks, gatherings and fundraising events throughout the year. However, raising awareness is a slow process, and the Irish Health Executive continues to turn to 'standard' opinion, and publishes guidelines based on such, discounting alternative modalities of diagnosis; it also discounts ILADS recommendations of longer treatment and combination treatments.

Some minimal progress has been made regarding the awareness of Lyme and tick-borne diseases among medical professionals and the general public. The Health Protection Surveillance Centre (HPSC) established a sub-committee in 2015 in Dublin, with its primary aim being to examine best practice in prevention and surveillance of Lyme disease and to develop strategies to undertake primary prevention in order to minimize harm caused by Lyme borreliosis in Ireland. The subcommittee includes representatives from the medical profession, the scientific community and patient advocacy. The HPSC ran a Lyme awareness event in 2016 and publishes information for both health practitioners and the general public on its website.

However, the guidelines once again come down on the side of the standard 'two-tier' testing, which misses over 50 per cent of Irish patients with Lyme and co-infections. They criticize the 'German labs', those with 'chronic fatigue' who are looking to Lyme as a possible explanation for their condition, and the possible usefulness of longer treatment. They refer back to the IDSA documents of 2006 and post-treatment Lyme disease syndrome. Many would question whether such editorial comments should be in a government document of such importance. A recent review in the Irish parliament initiated by Tick Talk and ministers from County Kerry, where Lyme is endemic, generated the standard presentation from the Irish prime minister, who read from a script stating that 'the two-tier test' is the gold standard in Ireland, and questioned whether there is such a thing as 'chronic Lyme'. So, from the mouths of politicians, the same mantra, and there is currently not much hope for Irish patients suffering from these treatable and curable conditions.

Of note, between 2006 and 2016 research was done on hepatitis C; and we now have cures for this infection. During this same time period not much has changed with Lyme. It is still said to be easy to diagnose, easy to treat, and if patients are still sick after a short course treatment, they should 'get over it' as all they have is post-treatment Lyme disease syndrome.

We are stuck in a tragic cycle of denial and anti-science. If patients are sick with an unknown diagnosis, and we can't figure it out, the medical community should acknowledge the patient experience and accept that they are ill and that we in the medical community do not have all of the answers. We should not attack the patients and label them with psychiatric conditions or fabricated medical conditions such as 'functional neurological disorders'. While not every patient with 'chronic fatigue' has chronic Lyme, some of them do. And when they respond to antibiotic treatment, practitioners should acknowledge they 'missed something' and advocate for better advances in our understanding of these conditions.

The challenge of Lyme in Ireland is no different from the challenges in many parts of North America and the EU. There are strong opinions on both sides of the IDSA/ILADS debate, very few doctors acknowledging that these patients have a 'real' illness, despite much clinical experience and patient feedback that the treatments using the ILADS guidelines have worked for many of them. What is needed is better research, together with less polarization of opinion. Knowledge of this condition is poor: we need better education of the public, primary care givers (GPs) and specialists. We need better diagnostics, and a better understanding of the complex interaction of infection, inflammation and autoimmunity that is at the heart of these very complex multi-system and multi-disease conditions.

Acknowledgement:
This chapter was reviewed by Ross Murtagh, student, MMUH, Ireland.

Chapter 16

From Lyme disease to crypto-infections

The story of tick-borne diseases in France

Dr Christian Perronne

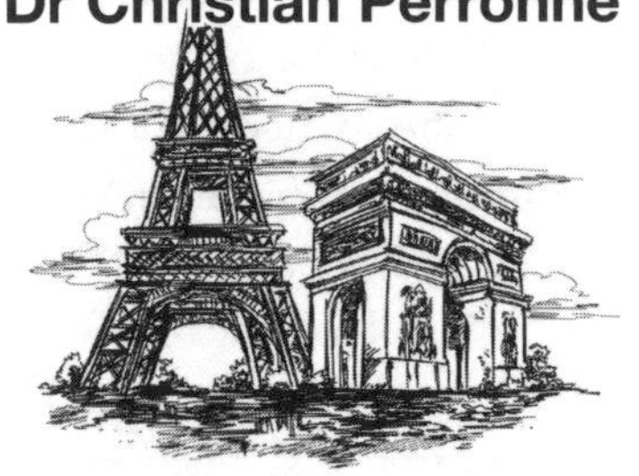

As in the whole of Europe, and most countries in the world, French health authorities have for decades followed the advice of experts under the control of a small group of leaders in the US belonging to the Infectious Diseases Society of America (IDSA), supported by the Centers for Disease Control and Prevention (CDC) in Atlanta, US. Recommendations from IDSA for diagnosis and treatment of Lyme and associated diseases are based on a very low level of evidence and are rather opinions of experts. In Europe, the European Union Concerted Action on Lyme Borreliosis (EUCALB) recommended the IDSA guidelines be followed.

Throughout Europe, including France, EUCALB made recommendations for the relevant medical societies and the National Reference Centers for Lyme Borreliosis. Recently, in 2017, the website of EUCALB disappeared. The group was replaced by an ESCMID (European Society of Clinical Microbiology and Infectious Diseases) Study Group for Lyme Borreliosis (ESGBOR).[116]

This organization did not allow any deviation from IDSA dogmas: Lyme disease is a rare condition, diagnosis is easy, serological tests are highly sensitive and specific, Western Blot is forbidden if the result of ELISA is negative, and antibiotic treatment of two to three weeks' duration allows all patients to be cured. Labs doing more sensitive tests were closed or condemned in court by legal action. Other effective tests, such as polymerase chain reaction (PCR), which allows the direct isolation of bacteria, are not authorized despite their current use in animals. In several countries, physicians treating Lyme patients for longer periods have been prosecuted and their medical licenses withdrawn.

Despite the fact that the persistence of Borrelia after several weeks or months of antibiotic treatment has been demonstrated, patients who have had the impudence to complain of persistent symptoms or of relapse after the end of a short treatment are classified as having 'post-treatment Lyme disease syndrome', suggesting that they suffer from sequelae, autoimmune disorders, laziness or psychosomatic disease. Thus, millions of people around the world continue to be rejected by the health system while suffering a high level of pain and fatigue, various multi-system signs and symptoms, become disabled and unable to work, get depressed, and maybe commit suicide or sometimes die silently at home.

Fortunately, as the IDSA guidelines are obsolete and do not fit with the Institute of Medicine standards (Institute of Medicine – IOM – of the National Academies, Washington DC), they were withdrawn from the National Guideline Clearinghouse (NGC) website. The NGC, funded by the Agency for Healthcare Research and Quality (US Department of Health and Human Services) harbored on its website alternative medical guidelines reviewed by IOM. However, in July 2018, funding of the NGC ended.[117]

Background

My personal experience of Lyme disease started in the early '80s during my internship in the Greater Paris University Hospitals (Assistance Publique – Hôpitaux de Paris). I used to work in an infectious and tropical disease department in the old Claude

Bernard Hospital, now demolished. At that time in Paris, there were only two hospitals dedicated to infectious diseases, the Claude Bernard and the Pasteur Institute Hospital. I met a young senior registrar, Dr Eric Dournon, who was working with the CDC to investigate a possible outbreak of nosocomial legionellosis in a Parisian hospital. It was a few years after the discovery of *Legionella pneumophila* during the famous outbreak that struck veterans during the American Legion convention in Philadelphia in 1976 and gave the infection its name. Dr Dournon learned from the CDC about the 'new emerging' disease called 'Lyme disease'. He worked in the lab to develop the culture of *Borrelia burgdorferi* and realized in France the first Lyme diagnostic tests based on serology.

Thanks to Dr Dournon, some patients could be diagnosed in France. He invited me to his office where he had posted on the wall a big table containing all the clinical and biological information about the first patients diagnosed with this 'new rare disease'. I was amazed and I learned a lot from him about the diversity of symptoms and many atypical forms of the disease. During my internship, I also worked in a rheumatology department in the Bichat Hospital. The head of the department was the famous Professor Marcel Francis Kahn, who was one of the major rheumatologists in France, a great specialist in autoimmune diseases. He knew Professor Stephen Malawista from Yale University, a discoverer of Lyme disease. Professor Kahn told me, at that time, that in the US, after the availability of the first Lyme serologies, some patients being treated for autoimmune diseases, such as lupus or rheumatoid arthritis, had been cured with antibiotics. I remember the story of a young American patient kept in confinement in a psychiatric ward for psychosis who was cured after one month of intravenous penicillin G treatment. It seemed that Lyme disease could be considered, like syphilis in its day, as the new 'great imitator'.

I was fascinated by these stories. After this early initiation into Lyme disease, I discovered, year by year, that real-life Lyme disease was not the same as the one described in articles or textbooks by the IDSA 'experts' or by my colleagues from infectious diseases, internal medicine, rheumatology, neurology or dermatology.

Pioneers in France

Meanwhile, Eric Dournon had created a National Reference Center for Lyme borreliosis and then became professor of infectious and tropical diseases in the Raymond Poincaré University Hospital in Garches, a Paris suburb. He was perfectly aware that Lyme serologies were not reliable and that became a problem. The poor sensitivity of serology testing was confirmed in several publications. Unfortunately, in 1992, Professor Dournon died at a relatively young age.

His National Reference Center was moved to the Pasteur Institute in Paris. In the Pasteur Institute, there was no expert on Borrelia, so the Center was subsumed into the leptospirosis lab. The reason for this was that both bacteria, although different, had a spiral shape! By chance, I was appointed in 1994 as a professor of infectious and tropical diseases in the Raymond Poincaré University Hospital in the position previously occupied by the late Professor Dournon, to be head of the infectious and tropical disease department. Unfortunately, when I arrived, the National Reference Center had already left my hospital two years previously. A few years later, microbiologists from Strasbourg in Alsace started a collaboration with the Pasteur Institute lab. Alsace is an eastern region considered to be an important hotspot for the epidemic of Lyme disease in France. In 2012, the National Reference Center was transferred to Strasbourg.

Garches is not far from Versailles, and parks and big forests surround this suburb. Consequently I saw far more Lyme patients than I had at my previous hospital located within central Paris. At that time, my main topics of research were antibiotic development, HIV/AIDS, tuberculosis, atypical mycobacteria and viral hepatitis. I was involved as principal investigator leading major national clinical trials on these topics. The number of Lyme patients increased in my consultations. A lot of patients with a typical presentation of the disease continued to have negative Lyme serologies. Seronegative Lyme cases, as proven by isolation of Borrelia by culture, had been described for years in the medical literature, including in major journals, so I was not really surprised.

The surprise came when I discovered that this presentation (symptoms with a positive culture but negative serology) was denied by the medical community, despite published data. Many patients complained of persistent symptoms or relapse after the end of treatment. Additional courses of antibiotics improved their condition. The first patient with severe seronegative chronic Lyme whom I cured had been very dynamic before becoming ill. He had been working full time as well as restoring an old house. When he became ill, he had experienced terrible fatigue and pain and problems with walking, and could hardly take care of himself day-to-day. He spent 15 years trying to understand what had happened to his health and to find help. He lost his job and his wife. People thought him lazy and depressed. He had seen around 80 physicians and 20 psychiatrists, without any result, before coming to see me. He was desperate.

Despite his negative Lyme serology, I thought it was worth trying an empiric antibiotic treatment as a diagnostic test, which is positive in case of improvement of the clinical condition with the treatment. After one month, he was like a new person. A few cases like this convinced me that there was a major public health problem. Later I took care of children who were in a severe condition. As their family doctors did not understand the origin of these children's clinical condition, parents were accused of ill treating them. Eventually, I cured these young people with antibiotics and they were able to return to a happy life with their beloved parents. I tried at that time to speak with colleagues about this major medical problem but nobody was interested in this 'rare disease'. At the end of the '90s, I was much involved in research, chaired several working groups to develop medical guidelines based on evidence and participated in several consensus conferences.

Fighting for acceptance

I was naïve and thought it would be easy to make rapid progress in the Lyme domain, as it was in other domains in the field of infectious diseases. For example, progress was rapid in HIV research. So I organized a meeting of different experts, including representatives of the National Reference Center for Lyme Borreliosis, which was, at that time, still located at the Pasteur Institute in Paris. I knew the Pasteur Institute researchers well, since I was vice-director of the National Reference Center for Tuberculosis within the Institute. I wanted to create a working group to design good research that would lead to the development of new, accurate diagnostic tests for Lyme or co-infections, and to design clinical trials for chronic Lyme cases. The answer of the chief of the Lyme Reference Center was: 'Chronic Lyme disease does not exist; patients claiming they have this are mentally ill or belong to a sect; physicians who treat them with prolonged courses of antibiotics are charlatans!' I was astonished. As he was not a physician and never saw patients, I asked him for his sources. He cited the 'experts' from the IDSA. Despite this amazing response, I continued to take care of Lyme patients, to increase my experience and to write research projects to get funding. I quickly saw that it was possible to get funds for HIV, tuberculosis or hepatitis C research, but impossible to get a cent for Lyme, a so-called 'imaginary' disease. I was shocked.

During this period, I discovered that some patients were joining action groups (Les Nymphéas and then France Lyme, SOS Lyme and Lyme Ethique). A website, Tiquatac, created by a patient treated and cured in the US by Dr Sam Donta, provided a lot of information for patients. Hearing from my patients that I was the only hospital specialist in France taking care of chronic

Lyme sufferers and improving their condition, these patient action groups asked me to help them. I accepted with enthusiasm. For me it was a shame and treason to the Hippocratic oath to abandon all these suffering patients. These early action groups have now been superseded by bigger and better organized ones. During the following years, very few of my hospital colleagues agreed to help me with the management of patients or with research.

In the early 2000s, some politicians (mayors, senators and deputies), alerted by patients in their region, and by the association Lyme Ethique, started to contact me. They were receiving many complaints from country-dwellers, huntsmen and forest workers who were being turned away by the health system. These politicians asked for a political debate. They sent messages to the Minister of Health. Thus the Ministry of Health asked the French High Council for Public Health (Haut Conseil de la Santé Publique, HCSP) to evaluate data about Lyme and associated diseases. At that time, I was President of the Communicable Disease Commission at the HCSP. Two reports were made, an initial one on prevention in 2010[118] and a second one on diagnosis and treatment in 2014.[119] Both reports are available, in French, on the HCSP website (hcsp.fr).

Narratives from around the world

Meanwhile, in 2010, I was invited to speak at the European meeting of the International Lyme and Associated Diseases Society (ILADS), organized in London. I discovered many physicians and scientists, mainly from North America and Europe, who had had exactly the same experience as mine and we were able to share useful information. Among them was Dr Richard Horowitz. Richard and I were amazed to discover that, despite there being an ocean between us and that we had never been in touch before, we had had the same experience. In France, I discovered a group of physicians, mainly general practitioners – the Chronimed group – who took care of many chronic Lyme patients and also of patients suffering from several chronic idiopathic (unexplained) diseases. They were following, as was I, the theories of Charles Nicolle who was a former Director of the Pasteur Institute in Tunis, Tunisia, and Nobel Prize winner in 1928. He postulated at that time that most chronic inflammatory or degenerative disorders had an infectious origin that could not be detected by the classical tools of microbiology. He created the concept of hidden infections (*'les infections inapparentes'*[120]). In the '50s, at the beginning of his career in Switzerland, before emigrating to the US, Willy Burgdorfer, the discoverer of *Borrelia burgdorferi*, the Lyme disease agent, and who was completely familiar with Charles Nicolle's works, published his findings on African borreliosis (relapsing fevers) and the concept of hidden infections, which he called 'occult infections'. Recently, in my book *La Vérité sur la Maladie de Lyme,*[121] I proposed calling them 'crypto-infections'. This term includes acute or chronic events, whatever the symptoms or the microbial agents involved in the disease process. Since these first descriptions of crypto-infections, several 'idiopathic diseases' have been found to have a bacterial cause, including Whipple disease (*Tropheryma whipplei*) and gastric ulcer (*Helicobacter pylori*). Ulcer was previously considered to be a psychosomatic, stress-related disease and the scientific community cruelly mocked the Australian discoverers of *Helicobacter pylori,* Robin Warren and Barry Marshall, before they won the Nobel Prize for Medicine for their achievement, in 2005. Physicians of the Chronimed group, who take care of many patients with crypto-infections, are supported by Professor Luc Montagnier, another Nobel Prize winner (in 2008) for the discovery of HIV.

As prevention of tick-borne diseases is not controversial, I participated in the first HCSP working group. A few years later, for the second working group on diagnosis and treatment, as President of the Commission, I asked not to be included in the working group to avoid any suspicion of intellectual conflict of interest. I could have been accused of influencing the group members. For the same reasons, the National Reference

Center was kept out of the group. In 2010, the first report on prevention and public education was released. I asked the health authorities for an information campaign directed at two groups: (1) populations at risk of tick-borne diseases (TBD) due to their professional, sporting or recreational activities; this involved installing posters at forest edges to inform people about the risks of tick bites, prevention of being bitten and how to remove ticks correctly if they did bite; and (2) physicians and pharmacists, asking them to put posters with photos of erythema migrans (EM – the initial cutaneous lesion or 'bullseye' rash, of Lyme disease, seen in around half of infected patients) in their waiting rooms and pharmacies. Unfortunately, the health authorities took no action. They told me that it was harmful to scare people and that it could have bad consequences for tourism.

In 2014, the second HCSP report on diagnostic methods and treatment options was released.[122] The working group was composed of hospital physicians, one of whom was looking after Lyme patients, a general practitioner taking care of Lyme patients, veterinarians, microbiologists, a sociologist and public health professionals. Professor Patrick Berche, who was Dean of the prestigious Faculty of Medicine Necker in Paris, and who is now Director of the Pasteur Institute of Lille, agreed to participate and did a great job. I was pleasantly surprised to read their report, since the major problems were raised. First of all, the report said that the calibration of serologic tests for Lyme was not adequate, making the tests unreliable in many cases. They underlined the great variability among commercial tests. The turnover of available tests was high, with many serology kits used a few years before no longer existing. The new tests were calibrated by comparing them with the older ones, without revisiting the methods to evaluate sensitivity and specificity. The report emphasized that 20 out of 33 ELISA tests for Borrelia, marketed in France, and four out of 13 Western Blot tests, were not reliable.

The report mentioned the fact that co-infections with other microbes are probably a frequent event, but that accurate diagnostic tools for these do not exist in routine clinical practice. It was underlined that patients suffering from multi-system symptoms with uncertain etiology could have chronic Lyme disease but also a disease linked to co-infections, reinforcing the concept of crypto-infection. Muriel Vayssier-Taussat, a researcher in a lab at the Maisons-Alfort School of Veterinary Medicine who worked on the microbes present in ticks, was a member of the working group. She presented her results, now published, about the presence of different species of Bartonella (including animal species) in the blood of patients suspected of suffering from chronic Lyme disease.[123] Thus, people suffering from an unidentified syndrome combining general signs (fatigue, pain, etc.) and involvement of several systems (neurologic, muscular-skeletal, cardiac, cutaneous, etc.) should be investigated to eliminate a differential diagnosis and should receive an empiric antibiotic treatment as a diagnostic test. These statements were very positive and represented a significant breakthrough in the Lyme polemic. However, this report did not succeed in influencing the specialist physicians and did not modify the view of medical societies, health insurers, the National Order of Physicians or the Ministry of Health.

At that time I published a review of the medical literature showing that routine diagnostic tests were not reliable.[124] The low sensitivity of Lyme serologies was then confirmed by a meta-analysis published in 2016.[125] A report from the European Centre for Disease Prevention and Control (ECDC), released on the ECDC website in April 2016, has confirmed that the serologic tests are not well calibrated. The main cause is that it is almost impossible to define populations of ill patients suffering from chronic Lyme for sure, and of healthy controls, some of them being infected without knowing it.[126]

The fight against physicians

The consequence was a counter-offensive and the persecution of physicians started after the publication of the 2014 HCSP report.[127] This witch hunting was a real paradox, given these attacks against doctors and pharmacists were not based on scientific findings. At that time, a French biologist from Strasbourg, Viviane Schaller, was sentenced by the courts to a suspended prison term and a fine of more than €200,000, because she performed more sensitive Western blot tests, as done in some German labs, even if the ELISA result was negative. Her lab was closed down. A pharmacist from Strasbourg, Bernard Christophe, who made an effective cocktail of herbs for the treatment of chronic Lyme patients who could not get access to antibiotics, was also sentenced. Patients were full of support for him, but he was found guilty though there were zero complaints against him. He told me, during the trial, that he could not endure the possibility that his grandchildren might think that he was a crook. He died of a heart attack, I assume due to the stress, three days before the verdict on appeal. During this period, medical licenses were withdrawn from several general practitioners, despite zero complaints from patients. Furthermore, during this black period, the government in February 2015 rejected a draft law recognizing chronic Lyme disease, supported by 70 deputies.

Lyme patients were up in arms throughout the country. Judith Albertat, a former Air France pilot, who was at that time President of Lyme Sans Frontières, a patient association, published a book on her story in 2012. She boosted the attention given to the issue by politicians. However, the impact of the action groups was relatively low. There were several associations of patients and supporters. They were working separately and were not well recognized by the authorities. They often used non-scientific arguments, which were not convincing. I worked with a small number of physicians and a PhD researcher in immunology, Hugues Gascan, to create a federation of the associations, including a scientific council of physicians and scientists, in order to make their actions stronger and more professional. The French Federation Against Tick-borne Diseases (FFMVT) was created in September 2015.[128] Three associations joined together with a collective of physicians and researchers with the slogan 'Patients Physicians Researchers Together'. A scientific council was created. Patients and colleagues asked me to chair this council and I accepted with pleasure. Dr Raouf Ghozzi, a hospital specialist in infectious diseases, working in Lannemezan in the Pyrenees, who is one of the rare hospital doctors to take care of Lyme patients, was elected President of the Federation. The creation of the federation FFMVT had a tremendously positive impact. Advocacy could be based on scientific arguments and medical literature, showing that evidence was on the side of the Federation. This transparency and scientific support dramatically increased the seriousness with which the media, politicians and health authorities considered the problem.

Lyme in the media

Before 2015, it was quite impossible to speak positively about chronic Lyme disease in the French media. I was aware of several reports that were blocked by the media directors. The first significant breakthrough was achieved by the journalist Chantal Perrin, who made a film about chronic Lyme disease but also about relapsing fever in Africa, another kind of borreliosis. In May 2014, she broadcast the film on the France TV5 channel at prime time. The film, *'Quand les tiques attaquent'*,[129] was very successful, with a huge audience. Since the film was translated into English ('The silent epidemic'), the national success was confirmed at the international level. Many television stations throughout the world broadcast it. It was very pleasing for Chantal, of course, but also for all the patients, since it facilitated the change of public opinion. Later on, Chantal Perrin published a book with Roger Lenglet, *L'Affaire de la Maladie de Lyme*.[130]

In France, several articles and broadcasts in various media followed the release of the film. A few months later, another successful report of a 'Special investigation', *'Lyme: l'épidémie invisible'* (Lyme: the invisible epidemic) was broadcast on Canal Plus TV.[131] It was put together by Bernard and Benjamin Nicolas.

Progressively, I observed a shift from 'health journalists' to 'social issues journalists' taking an interest, showing that awareness of this important public health issue was increasing. This shift enabled the publication of much more objective articles and reports. I realized at that time that a number of 'health journalists' habitually work with a network of physicians whom they have known for a long time and are on friendly terms with.

These advisors are usually influential professors of medicine or pharmacology, who apparently think that they know everything and who are reluctant to change or to discuss new ideas. It also appears that many journalists did not check the data in the medical literature themselves. The social issues journalists don't have such links with health professionals, having a more neutral approach. Several journalists read scientific published data, instead of listening to narrow-minded key opinion leaders. They also interviewed patients. They were amazed to discover so many people who had had their personal, family and professional lives destroyed by chronic Lyme disease and co-infections, sometimes for decades of serious disability. Many of the patients had been sent for psychiatric treatment. Journalists were convinced when these patients could relate their personal histories, tell how their lives had changed after finding a Lyme-literate medical doctor, and how their health had recovered after several months of anti-infection treatments.

These people suffering from crypto-infections were not hypochondriacs or suffering from imaginary symptoms; after their health improved they stopped complaining, smiled and once again took care of their families and returned to work. In 2016, major popular newspapers (Gwendoline Dos Santos in *Le Point*; Isabelle Léouffre in *Paris-Match*) published articles that included patient interviews. In July 2016, the Lyme cause made the front page of the famous weekly magazine *L'Obs*, with the title: '*Maladie de Lyme, l'épidémie qu'on vous cache. 100 médecins lancent l'alerte*' (Lyme disease, the epidemic that is hidden from you – 100 physicians sound the alarm). The article was written by Emmanuelle Anizon. In fact, 100 physicians (some of them from the Federation FFMVT) followed me, helped by the major contribution of Dr Raouf Ghozzi and Dr Thierry Medynski, and signed a petition, 'The appeal of the hundreds', asking for a political and medical change about Lyme and other tick-borne diseases. Corinne Eyot-Daures, secretary of the Federation, did a great job in contacting many professionals in a short time. This appeal on the front page of a major journal was a tremendous success. The number of copies sold was a record for that year. It was followed by an exponential increase in articles and broadcasts about Lyme disease.[132]

Building awareness

This media debate helped many physicians to hear about Lyme and associated diseases. Too many of them had not really heard about them before or had learned that Lyme was rare in France, easily diagnosed and easily treated without sequelae. The French Society of Infectious Diseases (Société de Pathologie Infectieuse de Langue Française, SPILF) and the French College of Professors of Infectious and Tropical Diseases (CMIT) which I had previously chaired over several years, appear to remain under the control of the National Reference Center for Lyme Borreliosis in Strasbourg, itself under the influence of IDSA, EUCALB and then the ESCMID group ESGBOR. They always referred to the consensus conference on Lyme borreliosis, organized by the SPILF in 2006, which was a mirror of the IDSA guidelines. They did not take into account the 2014 report of the French High Council for Public Health (Haut Conseil de la Santé Publique, HCSP). Despite this omerta, hundreds of French physicians, mainly general practitioners, would like to take care of patients suffering from chronic Lyme or other crypto-infections, but it appears they remain afraid of punitive sanctions, especially when the patient has a negative serology. Thus, it is very difficult for a French patient to find a Lyme-literate medical doctor. Apprently, most of the specialists and hospital physicians reject the idea of chronic Lyme and therefore reject the patients. Patient associations help them to find a doctor. Some French patients could have access to diagnosis with polymerase chain reaction (PCR) test for Borrelia or co-infections, performed in veterinary labs, but the authorities forbid this practice. At the European level, the consequence is a terrible situation for Lyme patients in many countries, especially in the UK and the Nordic countries. It appears access to treatment is completely impossible. In Germany, official guidelines are close to those of the rest of Europe.

However, German patients, thanks to a relatively independent private health system, are luckier. They can have access to more sensitive diagnostic tests and to prolonged anti-infection treatments. In Eastern European countries, there is more freedom since physicians and labs are less controlled. I discovered several years ago that ESCMID appeared to be under the influence of the IDSA Lyme group. In 2009, a French professor in infectious and tropical diseases organized, under the auspices of ESCMID, an international 'continuing medical education' course for doctors on zoonoses (human infections acquired from other animals). He was a friend and invited me to give a talk on Lyme disease. Physicians from many European countries attended the meeting. The audience was very interested by my talk and I received excellent feedback with good marks and comments from participants. My friend was also happy and told me that he appreciated my talk, which was well documented with a lot of scientific references. I was very surprised to discover, the year after, that he asked the Director of the French National Reference Center to give the lecture and deliver the IDSA dogmas.

Unreliable diagnostics

In June 2016, in parallel with the 'Appeal of the hundreds' starting legal action, a consortium of 150 (and later 200) patients took action against all the Lyme serology manufacturers for lack of information about the inaccuracy of their tests. In consequence, the French judges are asking manufacturers to provide arguments to prove that their serologic tests are valid – a difficult task for the manufacturers, when a published meta-analysis shows that they are not.[133] In 2019, trial instructions continue.

Just after this media storm, in September 2016, the health authorities, Minister of Health, Director General of Health and High Authority for Health (*Haute Autorité de Santé*, HAS) acknowledged that there is a big public health problem and that diagnostic tests and treatment strategies should be revised. The Minister of Health, Marisol Touraine, acknowledged publicly that many chronic Lyme patients are being abandoned and rejected by the health system, and she announced she was launching a National Plan against Lyme disease and other tick-borne diseases. In acknowledgment of the work conducted by my department to help chronic Lyme patients, the Minister decided to create a full-time position for a physician in my department to help me with the management of patients and to organize research. Professor Agnès Buzyn, who was president of the HAS (and who became Minister of Health in May 2017) facilitated the organization of an official working group to review the problem. For the first time, public funds were allocated for research. A research project looking at a national cohort of patients was planned.

During this period of turmoil, a fifth association of supporters, *Le Droit de Guérir*, was founded. In February 2017, a long-term neurology patient with paralysis and confined to a wheelchair was cured after three months of anti-infection treatment, which I had prescribed despite a negative Lyme serology result. Before treatment, she sent her blood to a veterinary lab and had to give the name of a dog (Mirza) to have her blood tested. The veterinary PCR test was positive for Borrelia. Thanks to the anti-infection treatment, she was able to take up skiing again a few months later. She lodged a complaint at the penal court 'against persons unknown', for 'aggravated deceit'.

A multi-disciplinary group of experts was set up at HAS, including representatives of medical societies, physicians from several specialties, microbiologists, general practitioners, the National Reference Center for Borreliosis, patients, Lyme-literate medical doctors and a PhD researcher from the Federation FFMVT. This was initially co-chaired by Professor Jérôme Salomon, who worked in my department. In January 2018, Jérôme Salomon was appointed Director General for Health at the Ministry of Health. The goal is to try to find a consensus for diagnosis and treatment. If this is not possible, the Federation has asked for two options to be accepted. The working group met for the first time in March 2017 and has produced Recommendations for Good Practice, made up of two texts – a short text of 'Recommendations' that is theoretically consensual and a long text which corresponds to a 'Review' and includes a bibliography. In the long text, differing opinions are expressed.[134]

For the clinical forms of Lyme disease, Lyme serology is recommended (the IDSA method of serology – i.e. the 'two-tier test' (page 65) – was added after the final consensus by some experts in the group, without the agreement of the others, who consider that this method is not evidence based.) The two-tier test is a serology by the ELISA method only. The second step, a serology by the Western Blot method, can be performed only if the ELISA result is positive. In fact, the important point in the final and published text is that a positive serology result is not mandatory to establish the diagnosis. The text defined (as in the previous 2014 report by the HCSP) a syndrome called SPPT (*syndrome polymorphe persistant après une possible piqûre de tique*) which means 'Persistent polymorphic syndrome possibly due to a tick bite'. This syndrome may be due to Lyme disease, co-infections and/or other factors. The link with a tick bite does not have to be established. Serology for Lyme or co-infections may be negative.

SPPT is close to the PTLDS (post-treatment Lyme disease syndrome) originally described by the IDSA. The difference is that for SPPT, there is no need for a proven Lyme diagnosis and no need for previous antibiotic treatment. These details are important since, when the term PTLDS was created, it originally referred to persistent signs and symptoms that were considered as not due to a possible persistent infection. So patients were sent to psychiatry or received another diagnosis than chronic Lyme disease.

In 2018, the possible causes of PTLDS include possible persistent bacterial infection. In cases of SPPT (persistent polymorphic syndrome possibly due to a tick bite), every general practitioner can prescribe, after exclusion of another diagnosis, an empiric antibiotic treatment, one month of doxycycline, used as a diagnostic test. A response to treatment confirms the bacterial origin. The initial response may be improvement but also worsening of signs and symptoms (the Herxheimer reaction). It is also possible to prescribe anti-infection drugs beyond one month, without limitations on the duration or on which drugs. The general practitioner must define the medical care with a clinical reference center (either a regional center or one of five national centers). Centers will be appointed by the Ministry of Health after a national call. Reference centers should have representatives of Lyme patients on their steering committee. Treatments and outcomes must be registered in order to collect data for research. Some volunteer patients will be included in clinical trials.

Reference centers will receive funds for manpower and material resources, in order to register the data. While waiting for the reference centers to be appointed and funded mid-2019, physicians can continue to prescribe as usual. The recommendations are to be regularly reviewed, at least every two years.

After the final agreement, colleagues who worked within the group, and agreed until the last meeting, refused to sign and launched attacks to obtain the support of medical societies. Several learned societies asked for a boycott of the text. As mentioned previously, some modifications to the text of the Recommendations were added by the French Infectious Disease Society (SPILF) and by the Lyme Borreliosis National Reference Center of Strasbourg (which were represented in the group), without the agreement of the members from the Federation FFMVT! Despite the attacks, the recommendations were officially released in July 2018 by the High Authority for Health, HAS (Haute Autorité de Santé).[135]

These new French recommendations do represent progress, but there is no guarantee at the time of writing (the beginning of 2019) that the reference centers will be established according to the recommendations (e.g. participation of patients and Lyme doctors). These recommendations triggered unprecedented violent and irrational attacks from the anti-Lyme lobbies, in the name of science but not based on science.

Advocacy efforts

Meanwhile, I agreed to chair the European conference of the International Lyme and Associated Diseases Society (ILADS) in Paris, 19-20 May 2017. This meeting was a great success. The number of participants for a European meeting of this organization was double that at previous meetings and the level of scientific communications was high. Some ILADS executives went to the French HAS to meet the working group on Lyme disease. The media coverage of chronic Lyme remains high, especially after the ILADS conference in Paris, and is continuing in 2019. The public debate is continuing to grow and some professions who are at risk, such as forest workers, are asking for action. Dr Philippe Raymond, a general practitioner and member of the Chronimed group, is now organizing continuing medical education about the management of chronic Lyme disease and co-infections throughout France.

During these two decades of fighting, my secretary Françoise Kostas has done a fantastic job helping me. Thanks to her, I have been able to make progress with the issues more efficiently.

In addition to my international involvement in ILADS, I have joined the Ad Hoc Committee for Health Equity in ICD11 Borreliosis Codes. The members of this committee represent highly skilled professionals from North America, the Asia-Pacific region, Africa, South America and Eastern, Western and Northern Europe; we are concerned with borreliosis infections that lead to human illness and are caused by multiple species of spirochetes from the *Borrelia burgdorferi sensu lato* complex and relapsing fever borreliosis distributed worldwide. Many members are scientific and medical experts and have worked on borreliosis for two or three decades, and between them have published many hundreds of peer-reviewed research papers and studies. They serve as leaders, clinicians and professors across numerous well-respected academic and research centers. We have members who are regularly consulted by the World Health Organization (WHO) and governments on the development of health systems, surveillance practices, patient-centered care, ageing, zoonosis and other specialized areas. Other members are experts in governance, accountability, institutional reform, climate change, capacity building and human rights. This Committee was formed to address a key obstacle to patient care – namely, the outdated International Classification of Diseases, or ICD, codes that are owned and developed by WHO. The ICD codes are used by most countries in the world to define and diagnose diseases and are a 'standard diagnostic tool for epidemiology, health management and clinical purposes'.

Treating Lyme disease globally

However, the current ICD codes (ICD version 10) for Lyme and relapsing fever borreliosis represent a very small number of the symptoms and complications common to these infections. We had meetings in Geneva at WHO and with United Nations (UN). In 2017 and 2018, we met two Special Rapporteurs of the UN. We published two reports, which helped to open these doors: *The Situation of Human Rights Defenders of Lyme and Relapsing Fever Borreliosis Patients* and *Updating ICD11 Borreliosis Diagnostic Codes* (see page 285).

They document how the absence of adequate diagnostic codes, the absence of reliable diagnostic tests and the rejection by physicians of millions of patients all around the world is no longer acceptable. The reports support the violation of human rights on all the continents. The WHO ICD10 recognized only four codes for Lyme disease, without any recognition of the numerous clinical forms, especially those linked to the chronicity of infection. For syphilis, the other 'great imitator' disease, the number of codes is high. In June 2018, the WHO released the stable version of ICD11 which added new codes for Lyme disease, including a code for Lyme dementia and a code for maternal-fetal transmission or congenital Lyme disease. The need for the code for congenital Lyme disease has since been disputed, creating an international demand to protect the code and recognize the life-threatening complications of transmission from mother to child.

WHO has recognized Lyme borreliosis as a multi-region 'disease of consequence' for decades. In August 2017, the European Centre for Disease Prevention and Control (ECDC) published an ECDC technical document, the ECDC Tool for the Prioritization of Infectious Disease Threats Handbook and Manual, that includes Lyme borreliosis among the 30 most threatening diseases of public health importance.[136] The time has come to stop discussing the issue and to act. Lives are at stake.

In 2018, good news arrived from the US. A Tick-borne Disease Working Group was organized by the US Department of Health and Human Services. Their Report to Congress was published on 14 November 2018.[137] This report recognizes the lack of good diagnostic tests, the absence of good clinical trials to evaluate treatments, the persistence of signs and symptoms, and the possibility of the persistence of bacteria. It insists on the fact that co-infections have been neglected and that we don't have good diagnostic tests for them. It also acknowledges that there has not been significant research for decades and asks to fund research. This report to Congress describes many issues the French national plan tried to address. Thus, France and the US follow closely related pathways that should lead to global recognition of chronic Lyme disease.

Speaking with Marie-Pierre Samitier, a television journalist and writer, about the Lyme saga, she pushed me to write a book on my experience. I followed her advice. In parallel, she wrote her own book, *Le Mystère Borrelia*. In January 2017, my book *La Vérité sur la Maladie de Lyme* (The Truth about Lyme Disease), was published in French by Odile Jacob Publishing, Paris.[138] It is an overview of Lyme disease, but also of the current abuse of the concept of 'evidence-based medicine'. Experts have forgotten that evidence-based medicine is a decision-making triad combining published data in the scientific literature, the clinical experience of the relevant physician and the patient's choice. For Lyme and associated diseases, the lack of funding for research, over several decades, has been responsible for a low or very low evidence base in the medical literature.

Grading of Recommendations Assessment, Development and Evaluation (GRADE) is a method of assessing the certainty in evidence. Over 100 organizations, including the WHO, have endorsed and/or are using GRADE to evaluate the quality of evidence and strength of health care recommendations.

According to the GRADE evaluation system, when the level of evidence in the research literature is so low, the experience of the physician is crucial, as is the informed consent of the patient who should evaluate the risk-benefit of the different options for the management of his/her disease.[139] The book reviews the Lyme disease saga, including the history, political issues, my personal experience, diagnostic tests and treatments. Co-infections are discussed. I explain why the name 'Lyme disease' is inappropriate and should be replaced by the concept of unexplained syndromes due to various hidden infections, which I call crypto-infections.

The first European Crypto-infections Conference is planned in Dublin, Ireland, for 31 May to 1 June 2019.

Chapter 17

Lyme and tick-borne disease in Spain

Dr Laura Alonso Canal

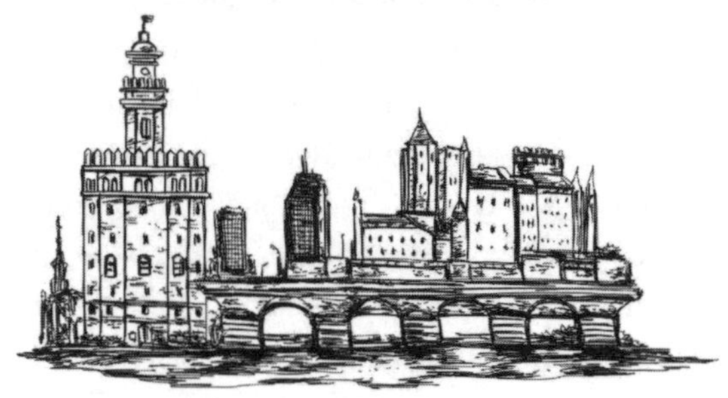

Here in Spain, it is said that Lyme disease is to be found 'only in the North, and is relatively uncommon'.[140] Though there is little epidemiological data regarding the prevalence of Lyme disease in different regions of Spain, very recently it has been admitted that the main vector of Lyme disease (the tick *Ixodes ricinus*) is widely distributed throughout most of the country. But even the presence of this vector is largely ignored by the medical community.[141, 142]

Most of our knowledge about tick-borne infections in Spain comes from tick-testing, rather than human testing. Up until quite recently, tick-testing performed by PCR (a way of detecting bacterial DNA in a particular sample) in laboratories here in Spain did not include checks for Lyme infection. Instead, research focused on other tick-borne diseases, such as *Rickettsia conorii* (Mediterranean spotted fever),[143] which is apparently significantly endemic in the center of Spain; Castilla la Mancha is in fact one of the highest endemic regions in all of Europe. Babesia is also very common on the Mediterranean coast and Balearic Islands, as well as in the North.[144] On some farms in the Balearic Islands, up to 80 per cent of ticks tested have been found to be infected with

Babesia.[145] Bartonella has also been found very frequently.[146]

The problem with these infections, as with Borrelia, is the high incidence of different bacterial strains. The Bartonella species most commonly found in the area around Barcelona are *Bartonella clarridgeiae* and *B. rochalimae*. The Babesia species most commonly found in the Balearic Islands include *Babesia caballi* and *vogeli*, as well as *thelaria, equi, annae* and *buffeli*. These strains are all known to be infective in mammals. If we are not even capable of diagnosing tick-borne infection in humans in our everyday clinical work, how can we be sure that people suffering from unknown illnesses don't in fact have such infections?

It's easy to joke that in Spain we are safe. Our ticks have been tamed. They have been taught not to travel south. They stay in the Basque Country or in Asturias (both northern regions) and do not bite humans, but stick to other mammals only. Unfortunately, however, my research and my own medical practice and experience have shown that this is not the case.

Both the general population and physicians are ignored when they speak out about the possible harm that a tick bite can trigger.

Though the number of reported tick bites continues to climb, people don't take care of these bites. They walk carelessly in the woods. If bitten by a tick, they simply remove it from their skin and don't consult a physician. If they do search for a doctor, sometimes this one removes the tick incorrectly (by spraying an antiseptic or analgesic compound on it before removing it, for example). Ticks should be carefully removed if possible with fine tweezers detaching the tick's mouth from our skin and never smashing the tick's body. Spraying any substance on the tick or burning it might cause the tick to 'spit out' more borrelia into our system. After tick removal, patients are generally told to just to go home and watch out for any possible symptoms. In the opinion of many of us who treat this disease, that is the wrong approach.

There are a lot of very good infectious disease doctors who are very highly qualified in Spain. I truly hope they will soon open up their minds to the existence of the tick-borne disease epidemic we have and the unreliable diagnostic tools that we are using.

There are some of us who work in other fields (I myself am a pediatric gastroenterologist with training in infectious and tropical diseases) or have a more alternative-medicine approach who have found this community of sick people to be fascinating to help and treat. Just a handful of them have already started treating chronic Lyme patients.

Infections are multi-systemic – that is, all organs and body systems are involved. General practitioners, internal medicine doctors, gastroenterologists, rheumatologists, psychiatrists, immunologists… these are just some of the specialists who are involved in the care of patients with Lyme disease and other multi-infection syndromes.

I have confidentially been told that over 50 per cent of ILADS (International Lyme and Associated Disease Society) doctors have had Lyme disease. Although I do not know if that affirmation is true, there is one thing I am sure of: it takes an unusual or personal reason for a 'regular hospital doctor' to drift away from the terrain of certainty and 'regular medicine' into the mists of uncertainty. Desperate chronically sick patients often require a more creative approach.

My family is from Galicia, a small square area just north of Portugal; it is a rainy region filled with good-hearted, humble people. It is also Lyme-endemic. People there just suffer in silence with pain, fatigue and autoimmune conditions, but in reality, much of the illness in the community can be linked back to tick-borne infection. Partly because of their humbleness, partly because of ignorance and lack of economic resources they do not complain. Galicians are said to have a rather 'sad and mournful' nature. As I have expanded my work in this field, I've often wondered how much of those personality traits could be linked to neurologic symptoms caused by tick-borne disease.

In the Basque country (the northern-most region of Spain) people are rapidly starting to act. They are closer to the French frontier, they have strong family links, and they usually have more economic resources than other regions in Spain. They are more eager to travel abroad for diagnosis/treatment or to go on a television show and denounce the situation.

When speaking with people who are living with these tick-borne conditions, I always tell them that I understand their fight; I understand their sense of unfairness. I am with them in their fight for answers. But I also tell them that science always advances slowly and that we have an optimal public social medicine system for which we should all be grateful. People in Spain with no resources whatsoever still have access to first class medicine, including the more expensive biologic treatments, million-dollar transplants and so on.

I sometimes even go as far as to say that we need to take responsibility for our own health as we are living at a time when everybody is getting chronically sick with conditions such as fibromyalgia, chronic fatigue syndrome, neurologic issues in children, autoimmune conditions… People in Spain are used to getting everything for free from the state, but there might come a time in our history where there won't be enough resources to give life-long pensions to all sick people because there are not enough healthy workers able to provide for this.

We must each try to find the easiest, least harmful and also cheapest way to recover our health, for our own wellbeing and for the good of others.

I do not want to frighten anybody but I also want them to be grateful for the sanitation system they have, and for the knowledge of the doctors who treat them; I want them to acknowledge that prevention is the most cost-effective thing to do and also to know that, sadly, they are not alone in their suffering. So many people suffer just like them, only they don't know that they have a multi-system infectious-disease syndrome. There is simply so much we still do not know. We must remain open-minded, humble and positive.

Chapter 18

Diagnosis and treatment of tick-borne disease in Germany

Zhaneta Misho

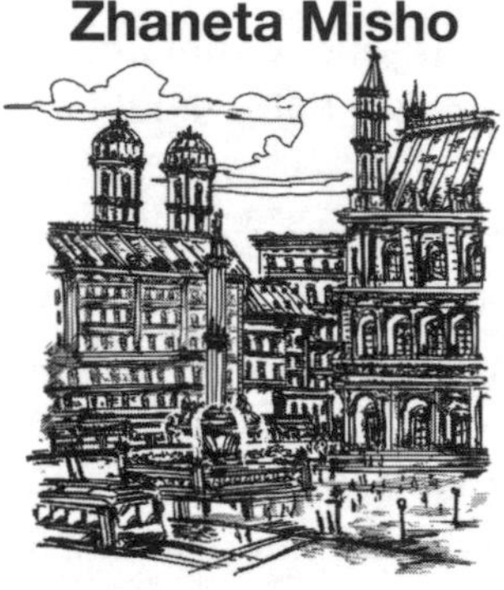

The first and foremost problem in the tick-borne disease field is to raise awareness that a patient's symptoms may be caused by an infection with a certain species of bacteria (spirochete), which was given the name *Borrelia burgdorferi* in 1982 in reference to Dr Willy Burgdorfer who first discovered it. It is predominantly transferred by tick bite, but occasionally as well by horseflies. It is only in the last decade that we have become aware of the impact and potentially wide dissemination of this problem. Already, back in 2010, Wolfgang Zöller, at the time Patient Commissioner to the German Federal Government, stated: 'Lyme-borreliosis belongs to the most underestimated and underrated diseases in Germany. In Germany about one million humans are affected.'

In Germany whole areas have been declared high risk zones for tick-bites with the associated development of Lyme disease. These have been identified especially in the south of Germany (Baden-Württemberg, especially in the Black Forest), eastern parts of Bavaria, recently moving north to affect South Hessen, parts of Rhineland Pfalz and Saxonia.[147] Zones with high incidence are found in other European countries as well, such as northern Switzerland, eastern Austria, the Czech Republic, Slovenia and western Hungary. And, since ticks become active after only a few consecutive warmer days (more than 7°C (44.6 °F)), the season in which one may get bitten stretches from late February to early December. There are frequent campaigns in newspapers and magazines about how to protect oneself and prevent being bitten and on the immediate appropriate actions to take in case of a bite. So general awareness has been raised considerably.

However, many bites go unnoticed and the first symptoms may appear to be just as innocent as a summer cold, but could turn into infections of joints, organs (including the eyes and the heart), meningitis or encephalitis. Symptoms in the long run are often not associated with a potential Borrelia infection. As has been discussed earlier in this book (the 'commonalities', page 12), these symptoms can include a wide variety of complaints such as: fatigue, depression, sleep disturbance, diffuse bodily pains, joint pains, food sensitives, chill and hot sensations, repeated headaches, discomfort in the throat and with digestion, loss of concentration and neurological deficits.

Many of these symptoms are usually treated with antibiotics, which often do help – but only in the short term. In the long run, our observations suggest that this is not a therapy option of lasting benefit. Sapi and colleagues (2011) have shown how the Borrelia spirochete can vary its form after antibiotic treatment, allowing it to persist for many years.[148]

Diagnosis

We are consequently increasingly alert to patients with the symptoms listed above. In such cases we test for *Borrelia burgdorferi* and other co-infections that have evolved recently. As we have seen earlier in this book, the big problem with all tests is the relatively high ratio of false-negative results. Besides the established ELISA test for Borrelia antibodies there are other methods, such as the Borrelia-Western Blot. A suitable screening test must allow for an increasing number of pleomorphic forms of the Borrelia spirochete; thankfully this is quite a dynamic field now. Thus, it is helpful to rely on a lab that has specialist experience with borreliosis testing. Our preferred partner in this respect is Arminlabs in Germany (www.arminlabs.com/en).

Besides the classical lab tests we use darkfield microscopy (magnification by 800 times, even up to 2000 times) to investigate a patient´s freshly drawn blood. In some cases, spirochetes can be spotted and even be directly seen in motion. And besides, darkfield images of living blood still yield valuable other information of the health status of a patient; so it is a useful tool anyhow.

Treatment

At times a spirochete infection seems just the last resort in accounting for a patient's failure to get better. But chronic disease, silent inflammation, toxins from the environment etc, all add up to weaken a patient´s immune system. Thus, the first treatment step is to reduce this load. Our range of therapy options includes:

- Detox (hydro-colon therapy and/or chelation therapy for flushing out heavy metals)
- Systemic hyperthermia (raising the core body temperature)
- Mitochondrial strengthening with biological infusions
- High dose vitamin C infusions
- Eliminating electromagnetic smog
- Nutritional changes and supplements
- Life-style changes and stress reduction
- Guided meditation to activate resources in the unconscious mind.

I will briefly elaborate on two of these therapy options: systemic hyperthermia and guided meditation. In our experience, both these instruments play an underestimated role in the orchestra of available therapy options.

Systemic hyperthermia

Body temperature is an important factor that seems generally to be underestimated in its potential. The regulation of body temperature is a mechanism that evolved in mammals over millions of years. Why is it that the body reacts with fever – raising core body temperature – when we have an infection? Would it really be wise to suppress this procedure only because it feels odd / unpleasant? We know nowadays that an upregulation of temperature is a boost to one´s immune system. Just to refer to one among many effects: Multhoff (2009) showed that natural killer cells – which form part of our immune system – are increased and activated with raised temperatures via generation of what are called 'HSP70 proteins' that stimulate the generation of NK-cells. A raised temperature further increases lymphatic drainage, decreases extracellular pressure thus allowing easier access by leucocytes into regions of interest, positively influencing hypoxic areas and pH levels. Last but not least, combining raised body temperature with biological infusions enhances their uptake and metabolism. Hyperthermia therefore enhances health in multiple ways: it helps in flushing out toxins, supports desired physiological functions and enhances a patient´s own immune response.[149]

There are various ways to induce hyperthermia. Active forms include 'pyrogenes', such as. infusions of mistletoe extracts; passive forms include regional or whole-body hyperthermia. In both cases, heat is induced non-invasively. In the first case, it is generated by an electromagnetic field, in the latter case, by water-filtered infrared lamps over a special bed. This second option is time consuming and may take over four hours. The treatment is systemic since the whole body is being heated and, through rectal temperature measurement, can easily be quality controlled.

A hyperthermia session needs to be closely coordinated with other therapies. Immediately preceding a session we enrich oxygenation, mostly with high-dose vitamin C infusions (25-40 g) and, according to the individual case, other biological infusions and mitochondrial supports.

In treating persistent Lyme disease we rely on moderate whole-body hyperthermia. Moderate means we aim at peak body temperatures of 38.5°C to maximum 39.5°C (101.3 to 103°F). This is the natural fever range and offers best results.

Extreme whole-body hyperthermia with temperatures beyond 400°C (104°F) does not seem appropriate, since it does not harm Borrelia spirochetes. These increasingly can be found in birds as well as mammals (*B. burgdorferi* and *B. bissettii* which have been known to cause Lyme-like illness in people in central and southern Europe (Newman et al, 2015)) and birds have body core temperatures of 40-42°C (104-107.6°C), which naturally is in the range we try to achieve with extreme whole-body temperature.[150]

The rationale for hyperthermia lies not in directly damaging the spirochetes but in enhancing the potency of conjoint therapies (by improving distribution and metabolism) and in boosting the innate and adaptive immune systems of the patient.

Hyperthermia treatments are given in about 3-5 fractions with a pause of three to four days in between. Sometimes, when patients live close to our office, we give them one session per week. A daily fraction is not recommended since cells build up protective heat shock proteins and it takes about 48 hours to denaturate them again. Thus, a follow up-session should not be too close to a preceding session. These heat shock proteins, by the way – namely HSP70 and HSP90, which partly migrate beyond the cell membrane – do play an important part in stimulating the immune system. For quality control we always measure body core temperature rectally and we monitor pulse and oxygenation during a session.

While patients may well be a bit exhausted during the last phase of such a session, even a short time afterwards they experience a positive regenerating effect.

Guided meditation to activate resources in the unconscious

It may sound odd at first, but every patient has an enormous reserve of often untapped resources in his or her own subconscious. While we may consciously control functions such as breathing pattern or pulse frequencies, other functions, especially in our immune system, seem out of our cognitive control. This is not entirely true, however, and even in the very first meditation session amazing effects can be experienced. Guided meditations are a technique to teach patients to start communicating with their own body, selected organs and even cells. We offer this in a brief series of 45 minute sessions over time, even at home with just an internet (Skype) connection.

'Biological therapy' implies a treatment will help the body to strengthen and heal itself. Our immune system works best in a state of so-called parasympathetic dominance; this is when we are truly relaxed. When stressful situations persist, functions like digestion, regeneration and healing cannot be maintained to their full potential. This needs to be addressed.

But the true potential is far beyond that. The objective is to enable a patient to recognize common characteristics between bodily malfunctions and themes in life. As often in lasting healing, a change in attitude occurs (and may eventually lead to changes in lifestyle as well). This is a process of feeling and sometimes daring to look into hidden or frightening topics.

It functions like a mirror for a patient's whole Self.

Concentrating purely on bodily functions seems old fashioned but is still a widespread approach. Biological treatments, however, to achieve their full potential must involve joint body / mind approaches.

Concluding remark

'Biological treatment' describes a portfolio of therapy options that have in common the aim of strengthening a patient's natural resources. It tries to offload harmful factors (toxins, stress etc) and to boost natural healing. The ratio of benefit to undesired side effects is extraordinarily high! Nobody can guarantee that each and every therapy option used may truly be needed in an individual case, but when measures call on natural healing at least no harm is done. Observations, however, and – more importantly – patient's own experiences, indicate that these approaches finally can end long odysseys of suffering and doctor shopping.

Lyme disease and other related chronic/persistent diseases, with their diverse symptoms and diagnostic challenges, are ideal candidates for biological treatments.

Chapter 19

A summary of the European situation and new testing Tickplex and ELISpot

Dr Armin Schwarzbach

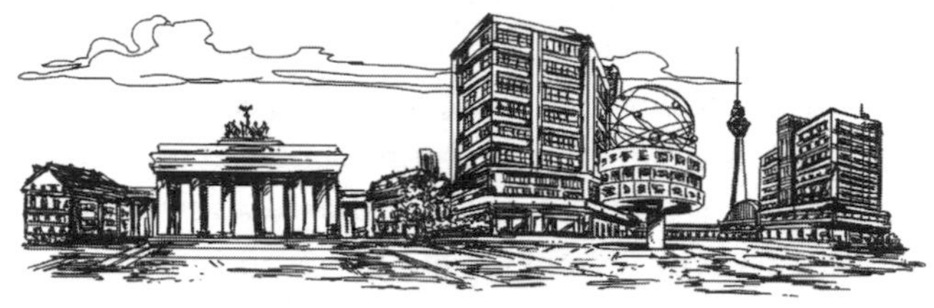

I am a clinical laboratory specialist, MD and PhD, and the founder of ArminLabs in Augsburg, Germany, which is highly specialized for modern testings of Lyme-borreliosis and co-infections. I have been serving as the international expert for the Chief Medical Officer´s Clinical Advisory Committee on Lyme Disease in Australia (CACLD) and as former director of the International Lyme and Associated Diseases Society (ILADS) in the US.

I am writing here about the European Lyme disease situation in my role as a clinical laboratory specialist working with patients to diagnose and treat Lyme-borreliosis and co-infections in over 50,000 cases in the last 20 years. In Europe, Lyme disease and co-infections are very often misdiagnosed and knowledge about tick-borne diseases seems be poor because of misleading guidelines. Nevertheless, many European doctors have contacted me in recent years to get support in the diagnosis and treatment of Lyme-borreliosis in their countries.

In 2018, members of the European Parliament called for the European Union to set out guidelines on Lyme disease because it is affecting between 650,000 and 850,000 Europeans every year. From European country to country, the diagnostic and treatment guidelines prove to be very different, forcing some sufferers to undertake a form of 'therapeutic wandering', crossing Europe to find solutions adapted to their infection.

As you have read already, Lyme-borreliosis is a bacterial infection by a spirochete named *Borrelia burgdorferi*, which can move everywhere around the body and be the reason for many symptoms and syndromes. It is named the 'known unknown' by Lyme-borreliosis specialists, a chameleon-like bacterium, difficult to diagnose and difficult to treat.

Lyme-borreliosis is the fastest growing vector-borne infection in Europe, as in the US. In Europe, up to 50 per cent of the ticks in Lyme-endemic areas are infected with *Borrelia burgdorferi*.

The problem begins with the fact that just fewer than 50 per cent of patients with Lyme-borreliosis recall a tick bite. Fewer than 50 per cent of patients recall any bullseye rash (Erythema migrans) as a typical sign of a fresh infection.

Without the recollection of a tick-bite or bullseye rash, chronic Lyme-borreliosis symptoms can be misdiagnosed as chronic fatique syndrome (CFS), fibromyalgia, rheumatoid arthritis, carpal tunnel-syndrome, Parkinson's, Alzheimer´s disease, multiple sclerosis, motor neuron disease, depression, autism and more.

European guidelines require doctors to use the Borrelia-ELISA for Borrelia antibodies as a screening test and not the Borrelia-Western Blot, even though the Western Blot has a higher test sensitivity (fewer false-negative results) and a higher specificity (fewer false-positive results).

The ELISA test, which is done at your doctor´s office, misses 35 to 60 per cent of culture-proven Lyme-borreliosis cases. The Western Blot identifies around 60 per cent of chronically infected patients, which means also a lot of false-negative Western Blot results in the case of chronic Lyme-borreliosis.

The actual laboratory tests for Borrelia-antibodies are not standardized and cannot exclude chronic Lyme-borreliosis.

In 2010, the European Union spent €1.1 million on the development of a 'highly sensitive and specific low-cost lab-on-a-chip system for Lyme diagnosis' by the Hilysens I Project. I have taken part as one of the scientific partners in the Hilysens I Project.

The good outcome of Hilysens I was to detect *Borrelia burgdorferi* antibodies against pleomorophic forms of the bacterium (L-Forms, round-bodies, cysts).

Based on this fact, Finnish University Professor Leona Gilbert developed an innovative test system to detect antibodies against these pleomorphic forms of *Borrelia burgdorferi* (the TickPlex system). There seem to be much better chances of finding positive Borrelia antibodies using the more sensitive Tickplex test system in chronic Lyme patients in the future.The TickPlex assay is performed on the basis of an ELISA. However, compared with other ELISA assays, this test contains a new antigen for round bodies/persister forms of Borrelia. TickPlex also allows for the simultaneous determination of multiple pathogens in the complexity of tick-borne infections with a high sensitivity of approximately 95 per cent and a specificity of 98 per cent.

TickPlex detects IgM and IgG antibodies of various bacterial and viral pathogens at the same time. It is the first ELISA system worldwide for all the main co-infections – Ehrlichia/Anaplasma, Babesia, Rickettsia and Bartonella – with much higher sensitivity to detect highly specific antibodies against co-infections.

Lyme-borreliosis does not only show humoral immune responses by antibodies, but can activate T-lymphocytes at the same time. Once *Borrelia burgdorferi* is not active anymore, the T-cellular immune response should cease.

It is not possible to test the treatment success based on Borrelia antibodies because the 'titer' of antibodies can persist in the blood for years. Recent *Borrelia burgdorferi* infections (e.g. 'bullseye rash' or 'summer flu') can develop antibodies after weeks and in around 40 per cent do not show them at all.

The Borrelia ELISpot can eliminate some problems. The test reflects the current activity of chronic and recent *Borrelia burgdorferi* infections. It is highly sensitive and can detect even one single *Borrelia burgdorferi*-reactive T-cell in the sample. With detection levels that can be as low as one cell in 100,000, this test is one of the most sensitive cellular assays available. It is between 20 and 200 times more sensitive than a conventional ELISA. It displays a similar sensitivity to a RT-PCR (Real Time PCR) analysis but detects the secreted protein instead of the mRNA (messenger RNA).

The ELISpot is a certified, externally controllable and standardized test, which can also be helpful when monitoring treatments. Results should usually be negative about four to eight weeks after completion of an effective therapy.

ELISpot, the 'new T-Cell Test' is a 'game changer' for Lyme disease. I quote: '... The sensitivity of ELISpot is estimated at 84 per cent, and the specificity is 94 per cent...' '... ElisSpot assays provide robust, highly reproducible data...' '... ELISpot can be retested for the acquisition of additional information in follow-up assays...' '... the two assay systems (ELISpot + CD57-cell count) complement each other in the quest to understand T-cell-mediated immunity in vivo...'[151]

Bernard Raxlen MD from NYC, the overall author of this book, found 95 per cent of his patients to be positive by Tickplex and 85 per cent positive by ELISpot tests last years. Both tests are extremely helpful in avoiding misdiagnosis of chronic Lyme borreliosis.

The average patient sees five doctors over nearly two years before being diagnosed with Lyme-borreliosis.

In Europe, doctors are forced to treat a chronic Lyme patient for a restricted time with antibiotics. The 'allowed' maximum is two to three weeks in general. If the patient is not cured within that time, they are designated to have 'post-Lyme disease syndrome' (PLDS), as you have read in earlier chapters; most patients are then treated symptomatically (that is, they are given drugs to suppress each symptom) and the persistent infection is not treated. Many of these patients develop psychiatric disorders.

Short treatment courses with antibiotics have resulted in a 40 per cent relapse rate, especially if the treatment is delayed.

There has never been a study demonstrating that two to three weeks of antibiotic treatment cures chronic Lyme-borreliosis. On the other hand, documentation is available demonstrating that short courses of antibiotic treatment fail to eradicate *Borrelia burgdorferi*. Records show that 40 per cent of Lyme patients end up with long-term health problems.

It is important to know and learn about each symptom that can be caused by *Borrelia burgdorferi* to make the right clinical diagnosis in time to start the necessary antibiotic treatment as soon as possible. The patient should be monitored by the doctor after being treated for any fresh infection, but especially during and after treatment of a chronic infection.

The socio-economic costs for all European countries regarding patients who are misdiagnosed or diagnosed too late can be exorbitantly high, as can the costs of treating symptoms with painkillers or immune-suppressive remedies like corticosteroids, with all their bad side effects.

The earlier you diagnose, the earlier you can treat a Lyme-borreliosis patient, and then the better the prognosis in general.

To summarize, with some proposals to improve this situation in Europe:

- Teach medical students about all Lyme-borreliosis symptoms in a standardized way and about problems with diagnostic tests and treatment options, including the long-term treatment aspect.
- Hold basic courses for GPs on the handling of tick-bites; symptomatology, including a patient's account of their medical history; problems with diagnostic tests; and treatment options for a patient, including long-term treatment with monitoring of the patient.
- Set up studies of: bacteria in ticks (tick-tests); improvement of diagnostic tests; and of long-term treatment and the development of new antibiotics against *Borrelia burgdorferi*.
- Run information campaigns for the European population on how to prevent tick bites and about symptoms in new and chronic infections.

Chapter 20

Tick-borne diseases in Australia – different things to different people

Dr Mualla McManus

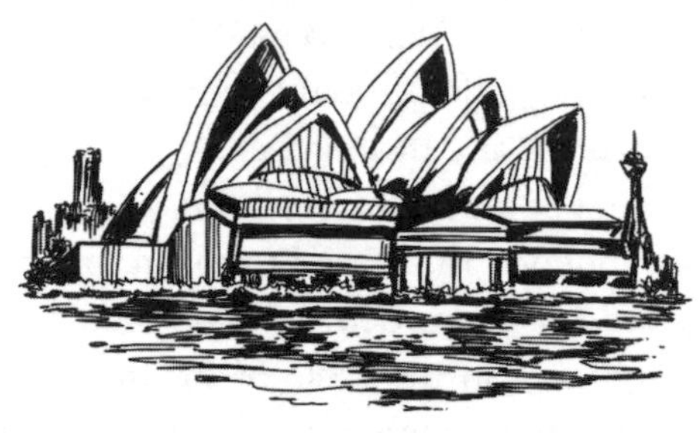

In Australia, many people self-diagnose with Lyme disease via the internet. Almost any chronic disease can be labeled as Lyme disease using such a limited approach. Moreover, through social media, Lyme disease is becoming a household term in Australia, despite scientific evidence precluding its existence based on the US East Coast definition of Lyme; this says the condition is specifically caused by the pathogen *Borrelia burgdorferi sensu lato*. *B. burgdorferi sensu stricto* has not (yet) been found in Australian ticks. Of course, overseas-acquired Lyme disease does exist in Australia. Australians are ardent travelers, particularly to the US, Asia, the Middle East, Africa, South America and Europe. Altogether, 9.2 million Australians travelled overseas between 2014 and 2015.[152]

The Australian story

It is perhaps not surprising that Australia has distinctive tick-borne disease pathogens. After all, kangaroos are not found outside of Australia and many animals are unique to other countries. The tick vectors are different in different parts of the world, so it should come as no surprise that Australian ticks and tick-borne pathogens are distinctively unique. The problem is that the Australian pathogens are yet to be conclusively identified although there is some antibody cross-reaction to Borrelia antigens (e.g. *B. burgdorferi* strain B31). Australia also has unique species of tick. Some have specific hosts like the kangaroo tick, echidna tick, etc.

However, with European settlement two species of ticks have been introduced into Australia. The cattle tick *Rhipicephalus (Boophilus) microplus* has come from Indonesia and *Haemophylus longicornus* from Japan (1902). In 2014, Barker and Walker updated Roberts (1970) *Source of Ticks in Australia*. They listed 16 species of tick that can feed on domestic animals and humans.[153]

For over 20 years Australian labs have been using the Lyme disease antibody test (based on strain B31) from the US to test Australians. This is based on assumed antibody cross-reaction between US and Australian Borrelia antigens. The situation is complex, leading to much confusion about the diagnosis of Lyme (or, more particularly, 'tick-borne') disease. The possibility that Australia might have European-related *B. burgdorferi* geno-species or, more likely, its own unique geno-species, has not been considered in the narrow medical view of Lyme disease in Australia.

In diagnosing the second recognized form of tick-borne disease, relapsing fever, blood film analysis is the accepted test. However, relapsing fever Borrelia species are only found in blood when the patient is having a relapse.[154]

Immune dysregulation is not part of assessing tick-borne disease in Australia, even though there is acceptance that the IgM/IgG ratios are relevant.[155] IgM is the first antibody response to pathogens. In a classic infection, after six weeks the antibody response switches to IgG. However, relapsing fever Borrelia infection continually induces IgM production without a switch to IgG. This occurs because relapsing fever membrane proteins change regularly so the host's immune system is fooled into thinking it is a new infection. Patients with chronic tick-borne diseases have continual IgM response without much IgG response. This observation can be interpreted in two different ways.

1. The immune system is dysregulated so Cd40 expression is required for antibody class switching.
2. The presence of relapsing fever Borrelia and co-infection prevents IgG production. Furthermore patients with tick-borne diseases usually make more IgG2 subtype which has less efficacy than IgG1.

In summary, the narrow view of tick-borne disease by Australian physicians and patients has hindered a professional approach to diagnosing tick-borne disease, and traditional physicians don't routinely do blood tests for relapsing fever. The almost exclusive emphasis on *B. burgdorferi* geno-species has led to major controversy concerning tick-borne diseases in Australia. This controversy was also fueled by the dominance of Lyme disease on the tick-borne diseases platform in the US. It may be that relapsing fever Borrelia is a more common and damaging tick-borne illness in Australia, but again one needs to be aware of the uniqueness of Australian Borrelia species that may not cross-react with European or other relapsing fever strains.

The recent discovery of a unique relapsing fever geno-species, *B. tachyglossi* in the Australian tick *Ixodes holocyclus*, and the echidna tick *Bothriocroton concolor* indicates that Australia does indeed have its own tick borne-disease pathogens.[156]

Historically, Borrelia sp has been documented in native wildlife (including kangaroos, bandicoots and other small marsupials) almost from the beginning of European settlement in Australia.[157] A relapsing Borrelia (*B. queenslandica*) was found in bush rats.[158]

The focus of Borrelia research in Australia up until the 1980s was largely on animal vectors, and the possibility of human infection was neglected. This changed with the recognition of human Lyme disease in Lyme, Connecticut, US. The first

Australian clinical case was documented in the Hunter Valley, New South Wales (NSW).[158] This was followed by the discovery of tick-borne illness on the south coast of NSW[160] and the central coast of NSW.[161] As is often found with Lyme disease, hallmark initial indications of disease in these patients were a bullseye rash, polyarthralgia (pain in many joints) and lassitude. The principal vector for Lyme Borrelia in temperate regions is the tick genus Ixodes (e.g. in the US, *Ixodes scapularis,* in Europe *Ixodes ricinus*). The major setback for study and treatment of Australian tick-borne disease was that Australian Ixodes ticks were not found to carry *B. burgdorferi sensu stricto.*[162]

The key medical research-supporting body, NHMRC (National Health and Medical Research Council), funded a major study (by the Westmead group) in 1989 to determine the existence of *B. burgdorferi sensu stricto* geno-species in Australia (the NHMRC study). This project led to the collection of 12,000 ticks from the east coast of Australia. Several different approaches were used to identify Borrelia species using in vitro culture, microscopy, and DNA techniques. Despite the fact that microscopy is used to identify relapsing fever Borrelia, the microscopy approach was inconclusive and so was abandoned. In vitro culturing was deemed unsuccessful. DNA techniques did not produce complete identification with Lyme Borrelia strain B31 sequences and so they were discounted given that DNA sequencing was in its infancy at the time.[163]

The paper by Russell et al (1995) describing these negative or inconclusive findings unfortunately cemented the dogma that Lyme disease does not exist in Australia. While this may be true for the absence of the *B. burgdorferi sensu stricto* geno-species, the symptomatic clinical evidence clearly pointed to a Lyme-like disease as a component of the Australian tick-borne disease spectrum.

For the next 15 years Australians became ill with myriad symptoms resembling chronic fatigue syndrome (CFS), polyarthritis, meningitis, encephalitis, myalgia encephalomyelitis

(ME), leaky gut syndrome and so on, with almost no attention being paid to the fact that some of the causative agents of these conditions (which occurred after a tick bite) might be tick-borne pathogens. Indeed, the fact that some of the patients presented with typical Lyme disease symptoms post tick bite was ignored, because the US diagnostic agents (based on strain B31) produced inconclusive results.

At about the same time as the Westmead group was conducting the large NHMRC study mentioned previously, Professor Richard Barry's research group at the University of Newcastle cultured Australian Borrelia spirochetes in vitro for short periods. DNA analysis revealed a *B. garinii*-like species with only minor changes in DNA sequence.[164] Professor Barry also instigated a clinical study, testing patients who were symptomatic post tick bite, which identified endemic regions in NSW, Manning River and the Northern Beaches. Later, Associate Professor Bernie Hudson et al published a paper about the culture of Borrelia from a patient bitten in Australia but who had travelled to Europe 17 months previously; the case was rejected as travel-related by peers (who followed the 'Lyme is not found in Australia' mantra).[165]

The findings by the University of Newcastle group clearly indicated the presence of Australian tick-borne pathogens, but they were overlooked in favor of the findings of the (negative) NHMRC study.

Not much happened until Karl McManus, my husband, became seriously ill with a tick-borne illness in 2007.

Karl's story

People who have been touched by tick-borne diseases are the ones who understand this hideous infection. In my case it was my husband, Karl McManus, who became ill after a tick bite in 2007. There followed a grueling battle, not only with multiple tick-borne infections, but also with an ignorant and indifferent medical fraternity.

Karl was working as a special-effects technician during the shooting of the popular TV program *Home and Away* in the bushy suburb of Terrey Hills in Sydney. Karl was bitten at night while working in July 2007. He came home and removed the tick by pouring kerosene on it. This illustrates lack of education about the dangers of tick bites and how not to remove ticks, in Australia at the time. A week after he was bitten he developed 'flu-like symptoms. Lack of education prevented early diagnosis of his condition. A week later we went on a five-week holiday to Europe. While on holiday Karl was developing more symptoms, but they were assumed to be due to jet lag. Upon landing in Australia five weeks later, symptoms of neuro-borreliosis, such as muscle twitching and extreme fatigue, became apparent, although we were not aware of that at the time. Each physician consulted (more than 50) was ignorant and not able to help. It took nine months to reach the conclusion that what he had was neuro-borreliosis. The infection in his dorsal root ganglion cells, or infection in the spine and cerebrospinal fluid, disseminated and his condition worsened. Karl suffered at the hands of ignorant physicians trying to put him into various diagnostic boxes of diseases they were familiar with, such as motor neuron disease, ignoring his obvious pathology of polyneuritis and poly-radiculoneuritis, or inflammation of spinal nerves. After three years of suffering he passed away in 2010. During his illness, we planned to work together to make tick-borne infections part of mainstream medicine.

Changes in the Australian Government's attitude to tick-borne disease

It was the passing of Karl that reactivated the tick-borne diseases issues in Australia. Earlier in 2009, Karl and I had formed the LDAA (Lyme Disease Association of Australia) and upon his passing I formed the Karl McManus Foundation (KMF) in his memory and continued to raise awareness (www.kmf.org.au). Then recently, in July 2017, the Karl McManus Institute was formed to concentrate on research. Both charitable organizations are Karl's legacy. The Foundation brought credibility to tick-borne diseases both by raising awareness and funding research.

Since 2010, because of Karl, there has been increased testing for Lyme disease in Australia. In 2013, Communicable Diseases Network Australia (CDNA) inquired as to whether Lyme disease should be included in the notifiable diseases list. Unfortunately, CDNA was referring to overseas-acquired Lyme disease. The number of positive results for overseas-acquired Lyme disease from Medicare labs had been very small over the previous 20 years and so Lyme disease was not included in the notifiable disease list in Australia (unlike the situation in US and Europe). Tick-borne disease caused by indigenous Borrelia continued to be invisible.

The KMF initiated the first Lyme disease appeal in Australia in 2011. The appeal enabled the distribution of brochures on ticks and tick bites to 2500 pharmacies around Australia. For the first time, Australians received tick-bite prevention advice and information about the infections ticks can transmit. The KMF Lyme disease appeal also led to widespread media coverage on TV, as well as in newspapers and magazines. The KMF has continued to raise awareness. Recent showing of Australia's first TV commercial about the dangers of tick bites is another example.

In 2012, the KMF instigated a meeting with the Chief Medical Officer of Australia, Professor Chris Baggoley, which led to the formation of the CACLD – the Clinical Advisory Committee on Lyme Disease.[166] The terms of reference for the CACLD were to report to the CMO on:

a) the extent of evidence of Borrelia spp in Australia
b) the best practices in diagnostics
c) the most appropriate treatment
d) the best way to educate the public and health professionals
e) research needs
f) further investigations that may be needed.

The CACLD commissioned a scoping study to explore research questions that need to be investigated in order to establish the presence or absence of Lyme disease in Australia. The scoping study established the extent of research that was needed to bring Lyme disease (if it existed) into mainstream medicine.[167]

The CACLD was dissolved in 2014, leaving more questions than answers. There was an attempt to understand the clinical side of the story by having a round table discussion with specialists from various disciplines, including psychiatrists, infectious disease specialists, cardiologists and general practitioners involved in treating current tick-borne disease. This meeting raised questions concerning clinical research and the validity of current treatment protocols.

Diagnosis and treatment of tick-borne diseases in Australia continued to be neglected until finally lobbying led to definite action by politicians.[168] This resulted in the Senate Enquiry, the terms of reference of which focused on patient needs, including the epidemiology of Lyme-like illness, and ways to reduce the stigma of Lyme disease, which had become a dirty word here. Patients were often ostracized, considered to be mentally ill and/or imagining their symptoms. In addition to patient needs, diagnosis and current research into the disease in Australia were listed in the terms of reference.

The Senate Committee accepted submissions from the public, health and research professionals and institutions involved. There were around 1200 submissions. The KMF submitted a detailed report on the unhelpful definition of tick-borne disease in Australia as Lyme disease, and the controversy resulting from persistent use of the Lyme terminology.

There were also senate committee forums where relevant individuals and institutions had an opportunity to personally brief Senators driving the issue in parliament. KMF representatives were present at these parliamentary enquiries.

The KMF presented the view that Lyme Borrelia is a small subset of *B. burgdorferi sensu lato* group and that in Australia we need to look outside the *B. burgdorferi* group, and especially consider relapsing fever Borrelia. As I have said, most people in Australia who think they have Lyme disease do not have the condition as narrowly defined by the CDC US tests, but their symptoms indicate exposure to Borrelia. It may be possible that a significant part of Australian tick-borne illness is actually relapsing fever or a unique Australian Borrelia group. In the early stages of infection, the clinical symptoms of relapsing fever and Lyme disease are similar,[169] although relapsing fever does not classically produce an erythema migrans rash. Recent sequencing of *B. tachyglossi* indicates Australian Borrelia can be hybrid geno-species, in that they consist of a *B. burgdorferi* group, relapsing fever and reptilian Borrelia. This may explain some patients having bullseye rash and the neurological symptoms from relapsing fever.[170]

Following the Senate Committee's final report, continued lobbying led to the tabling of the report in Parliament. KMF representatives visited Canberra and met with the Health Minister's team. The significant sum of $3 million has been set aside for research into tick-borne diseases in Australia. It was originally allocated for research into 'debilitating symptom complexes attributed to ticks' (DSCATT) in November 2017, and in January of 2019 successful recipients were notified. Murdoch University Group in Perth received $1.9 million, and the University of Melbourne group received $1.1 million. This funding is for five years. The outcomes of this research will hopefully establish tick-borne diseases in mainstream medicine. This funding is being coordinated by NHMRC.[171] It is a sign that perhaps the unhelpful focus on Lyme disease is changing; a new terminology surrounds this research funding, which concerns DSCATT. The KMF has also been representing Australia in the Ad Hoc Committee lobbying the WHO to update the ICD codes for relapsing fever and Lyme disease. In 2017 and 2018 the Ad Hoc committee on recognition of Lyme Disease/Relapsing fever – consisting of multinational representatives, including one from Australia (myself, Dr McManus) – met with special rapporteurs from the UN (United Nations) and WHO (World Health Organization) representatives to lobby for changes to ICD codes (International Classification of Disease). Every 10 years WHO updates the ICD codes. In 2018 ICD11 codes were to be adopted, so by lobbying the WHO and UN the Ad Hoc Committee managed to add to the Lyme-borreliosis codes, a code for congenital transmission. However, this success was short lived. The Canadian government lobbied to withdraw the code for congenital transmission of Lyme-borreliosis. This is despite CDC recognizing congenital transmission of relapsing fever.[172] However, I have been involved in updating the ICD11 code for tick-borne relapsing fever so that relapsing fever diagnosis becomes easier.

So some progress has been made, although the way forward is slow-paced and needs continual pressure from all stakeholders. Unfortunately, infection caused by *B. burgdorferi sensu stricto* (which is still yet to be found in Australia in 2019) still often dominates the discussion. Most Australians are not diagnosed at the time of a tick bite, due to unfamiliarity with early signs and symptoms of this disease by the medical profession and the public. The public at large is generally ignorant of the seriousness and danger of tick bites. Patient advocate groups continue to use the term 'Lyme disease', while others insist that there is no Lyme disease in Australia, thereby exacerbating the controversy.

Patient-doctor experience

Patients have difficulty finding doctors who will treat tick-borne illness. In the period between 2011 and 2013, there were close to 300 doctors across Australia prepared to diagnose tick-borne infections. Medical practitioners were developing an awareness of, and interest in, a new zoonotic disease in Australia. The KMF hosted three Australian tick-borne disease conferences between 2013 and 2015; dialogue with the department of health and the health minister by KMF resulted in a tender to the federal health department to educate the public and healthcare practitioners. The successful tender had to consult with all stakeholders, and closed on 15 March 2019. This work broadened the perspective of holistic, integrative doctors who were already treating chronic diseases. Patients who had previously been unable to get help experienced a reduction in their pain and suffering because they had attentive medical supervision.

A number of general practitioners have become members of the International Lyme and Associated Diseases Society (ILADS) and have attended conferences and training from ILADS doctors. The KMF has provided travelling fellowships for two doctors to attend the ILADS conference and get training with an ILADS educator.

But as the term 'Lyme disease' continued to be pushed by patient advocate organisations and the media, polarization and politicization have resulted, with many health practitioners becoming concerned about their medical board registration. Many practitioners stopped treating, while others treated cautiously. The situation became very serious for patients, some of whom have even been turned away from hospitals. Diagnosis of a somatic condition or 'conversion disorder' by psychiatrists has become commonplace. Today, more and more patients are resorting to being treated by naturopaths as most doctors refuse to help them.

There are only a small number of doctors still treating patients with tick-borne disease in Australia and these doctors have long waiting lists, which often means treatment gets delayed. Patients may need to travel long distances (more than 100 km) to find a sympathetic medical consultation. This is an unacceptable situation for a relatively common medical complaint that has serious consequences if treatment is delayed. Patients indicate that they have consulted up to 50 general practitioners and specialists before they have achieved a satisfactory diagnosis and treatment plan.

The upshot of the unsatisfactory situation in Australia is that many patients travel overseas to such destinations as Cyprus, Germany and Malaysia, seeking help. This can result in unacceptable and financially disastrous situations for the individuals involved and their families. Some have sold their homes in order to finance their overseas treatment. The overseas destinations can also exploit the vulnerability of these patients, as most don't understand Australian tick-borne diseases. Many who return from overseas for treatment do relapse after a short period of wellness or don't benefit from treatment at all.

Attitude of doctors to tick-borne disease in Australia

Most general practitioners in areas where ticks occur are aware of tick-borne diseases, but they are often focused on Lyme disease and miss the multi-pathogenicity of this problem. Many refuse to treat patients, some because they are afraid of their professional registration being compromised. Patients or doctors who are against tick-borne disease have complained to medical boards about minor medical inconsistencies. Medical registration bodies have used these complaints to treat these doctors unfairly. Most don't know how to treat because they are not sufficiently familiar with the signs and symptoms to make differential diagnoses. Infectious disease specialists (IDSs) have a better understanding, but patients need to be referred to specialists by general practitioners (GPs). If GPs don't differentially diagnose tick-borne diseases, IDSs don't get to see the TBD patients.

When patients mention Lyme disease to specialists like neurologists, cardiologists and rheumatologists, the response is generally very negative. However, if patients list their symptoms they get a better response. Australian tick-borne diseases usually present with complex symptoms with a propensity for more neurological as opposed to arthritic (Lyme) symptoms. Neurologists often diagnose patients as having a neurodegenerative disease (e.g. multiple sclerosis, motor neuron disease or dementia) without realizing that the symptoms can be due to tick-borne pathogens.

As I have said, many of the problems that the medical profession has with tick-borne disease in Australia originate from a narrow focus on Lyme disease and on diagnostic tests for the US *B. burgdorferi* strain B31, which cross reacts poorly with Australian isolates. Many doctors have been intimidated by this narrow focus on a diagnostic test for a foreign organism, and those who have sought to address the complexity of the symptoms have been subjected to untoward harassment from their profession. This situation is reminiscent of the treatment of tick-borne disease elsewhere around the world, but the Australian situation is undoubtedly one of the most extreme and unfriendly environments for medical professionals. It is time that things changed because patients are suffering.

The way forward is dialogue and research to guide the path of understanding tick-borne diseases and applying these findings to prevent, diagnose and treat them appropriately.

Chapter 21

Return to the Americas – Lyme in Canada

Dr Jennifer Armstrong

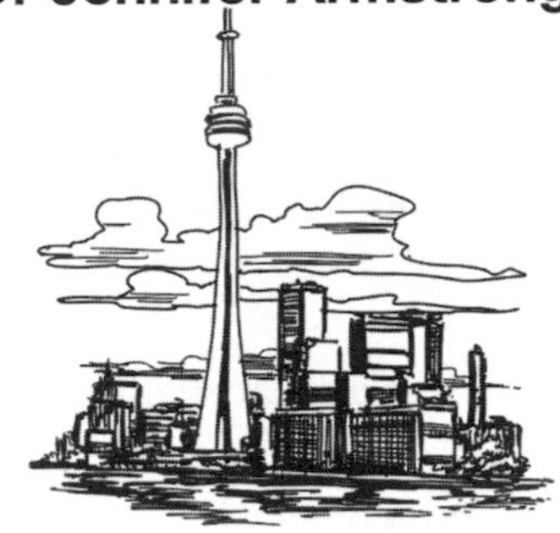

We have been seeing Lyme for some time in my part of the world. My first patient actually goes back to 1986, in Niagara Falls. After one month on intravenous antibiotics (Rocephin) her arthritis went away completely, but then returned. Being young and inexperienced at the time, I did not know what to do when her arthritis came back. As so many patients are, she was sent to the big city of Toronto to consult a specialist and was told she had post-infectious Lyme and that nothing more could be done. I often wonder how she is doing now; she was a young mother who was triggered to become ill right after her pregnancy. Being in Niagara Falls, Canada, we were right across the river from Niagara Falls, Buffalo, US. It is likely Lyme was already present in that area.

After that first patient, I moved to Ottawa, and trained in environmental medicine. All of our patients were complex. Most of them recovered when we helped them with food allergies, chemical sensitivities and metal toxicity. But some patients even with this help were unable to get better. We soon figured out that these were patients with Lyme and other vector-related co-infections.

It seemed, as the years went by, that there were more and more patients with vector-borne illness. It felt like 50 per cent of our practice, if we let it, could be helping Lyme-related patients.

If these 'Lyme' patients were able to get treatment they could get much better. The disturbing fact was that very few physicians had any idea about how to look for vector-borne illness or what to do about it. Ontario now recognizes that Lyme exists, but there is little education given to the doctors on how to look for chronic Lyme or for Bartonella or Babesia which are some of the co-infections. A tick bite is treated with two doxycycline pills in the emergency room.

If we do a battery of the tests available from our Public Health Lab (PHL – the main lab we use for testing) on these patients, often we see positive results for Q-fever, Rocky Mountain spotted fever (RMSFH – a rickettsial disease) and Bartonella, but the Lyme test is often negative despite all the clinical signs being present; this is because our Lyme testing is a 'two-tier' test starting with IFA (immuno-florescent antibody) testing – the first tier, which is often negative, prevents the lab from going on to the more important IgG, IgM second-tier test. There are many reasons for a negative test which are discussed elsewhere in this book.

Even with a positive first-tier test, the infectious disease specialists have not been supportive, or aware of the need to use intravenous antibiotics in patients who have neurological symptoms; thus it is very difficult in Ontario, Canada, to get an indwelling intravenous line, sometimes called a PICC (periferally inserted central catheter), put in. The gate keepers for having PICC lines, or portacaths ('Ports'), put in are the infectious disease doctors, and they typically refuse to believe Lyme exists unless their own testing is positive, which it rarely is, due to the very poor testing method. We are then stuck with using either oral antibiotics or herbs for treatment when we get a positive Igenex test, ELISpot test or make a clinical diagnosis, and it is very hard to get a very ill patient better on oral antibiotics.

Ironically, if we do have a positive first-tier IFA result from the Public Health Lab, the lab calls us to see what we have done to treat the patient. They keep calling until they know the patient is being treated. They are very concerned, but there is an obvious disconnect between Public Health, education and infectious disease doctors, or any doctor who sees these patients. If a patient does not have a positive lab result, then they are left to think that all they need is an SSRI antidepressant.

Of course, it is still useful to look at the total load of gut problems, food allergies, chemical toxicities and metal toxicities, to enable better and more achievable optimum health in these patients.

If there is any kind of mental illness exhibited by the patient, then it is wise to seek help from a psychiatrist. If the patient is bad enough to end up being admitted, then the 'team' of doctors looking after them on a psychiatric ward tends to ignore any other possible physical diagnosis, such as Lyme, even if it is diagnosed by Igenex, a lab in the US which is well known for its Lyme testing. This lab is more thorough and able to include more significant Lyme testing protein bands which are included in the testing. Unfortunately, in the basic US/Canadian testing the important bands for Lyme serology were removed when the Lyme vaccine was experimented with and when the vaccine did not work the significant bands were removed, in case any vaccinated patients ended up with a positive result for the wrong reasons. A psychiatric ward may then use the poor Lyme test and if the result is negative (inappropriately) tell the patient: 'See, you do not have Lyme', not understanding the science behind Lyme, and totally cutting out any family doctor who has been working with that patient prior to admission and who understands better how to diagnose and treat Lyme. Thus the patient becomes lost to follow-up, and likely has lost their chance to recover. Also other doctors in our country, including infectious disease doctors, are quick to label a complicated Lyme patient with a simple diagnosis like mental illness, as it is easy to treat with one pill. This is seen many times, with lack of understanding of the complexity of the symptoms, and also inappropriately placed sympathy, telling the patient it would be far better if they admitted that they had a psychiatric diagnosis.

If this sounds glum, it is. There needs to be much more education in Ontario, and likely all of Canada, on Lyme. Likely there have been unnecessary suicides among these patients when they feel so unwell and are only offered a 'Band Aid'.

Chapter 22

Lyme in Mexico

Dr Omar Morales

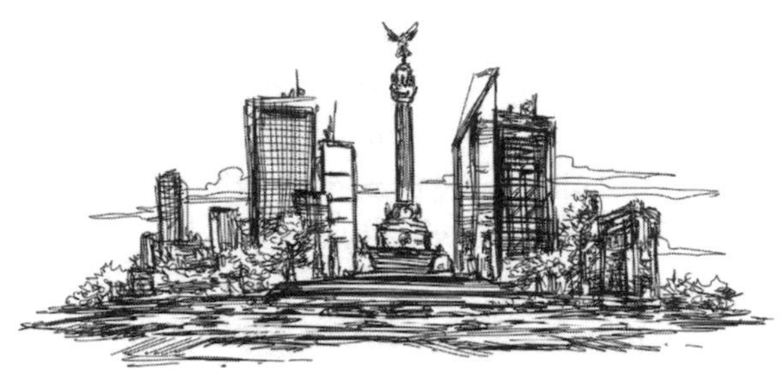

When you do a quick search on the web for the phrase 'misdiagnosed disease', it is no surprise that Lyme disease appears at the top of the results. However, if you conduct the search in Spanish, you find it to be very different – Lyme disease is nowhere to be found. This is, in part, due to the lack of information and understanding about the presence of Lyme disease throughout my beautiful country. Another reason for this deficit in awareness could possibly be the geographical variables (i.e. climate, flora and fauna) as well as the relatively short amount of time that Lyme has actually existed in Mexico.

Mexico has only recently become aware of its tick-borne disorders (TBD), which we believe are possibly the result of migration from the ancestral origins of Borrelia, or at least the origins that have been documented relative to these infections long ago. There are many interesting theories regarding the origin of TBD, ranging from the early ninth century in Europe to the Ancient Egyptian civilization to even a hidden biological lab at the end of the '50s. The oldest documented finding of the *Borrelia burgdorferi* spirochete was in Ötzi, a 5300-year-old ice mummy from the Italian Alps.[173] Whatever the actual origin may be,

I will not go into much detail on this topic in this chapter even though it is interesting. I will, however, state my view – based on information researched throughout my years as a Mexican/American physician – that it may be safely concluded, almost to a certainty, that Lyme did not originate in Mexico. Thus, though we are precariously behind in our 'Lyme consciousness', we began the race late, have fewer reports and data available, fewer infected people, less to say about the issue and consequently less awareness of the multiple problems that matter relative to this disease.

On the other hand, despite our 'delayed awareness', we have received worldwide accolades for our research and development capabilities in the area of tropical and zoonotic diseases, which fall within the Lyme disease domain. It is indisputable that 'Lyme disease' is actually a broad catch-all phrase for Borrelia infection together with its many co-infections: Babesia (32 per cent), Bartonella (28 per cent), ehrlichiosis (15 per cent), Mycoplasma (15 per cent), Rocky Mountain spotted fever (6 per cent), Anaplasma (4 per cent), and tularemia (1 per cent).[174] The percentages represent the proportion of the diseases that co-exist with the Lyme (Borrelia) infection. However, these may be higher than previously reported as other studies have shown up to 78 per cent of Bartonella found in Lyme cases, indicating that the incidence of co-infections is on the rise. Patients typically receive one or more co-infections from the bite of a single tick. Diagnosis of these co-infections remains difficult, and treatments for co-infections are often quite different from the treatment for the Borrelia (Lyme) infection. Sometimes a co-infection is only suspected when the patient does not respond well to his/her treatment for Lyme.

Babesia, for instance, with the highest co-infection rate, is considered a tropical disease and is not well known or studied in the US. It displays similar symptoms to malaria and is treated accordingly. Mexican doctors arguably are vastly better equipped to handle occurrences of malaria, parasitic infections and zoonotic diseases spread by mosquitoes than their northern US counterparts who are not called upon very often to treat these tropical illnesses. However, Babesia is becoming a more and more urgent issue as it is beginning to be detected in increasing numbers in blood banks worldwide.

Entry to Lyme

It was actually through Babesia that I originally got involved in treating tick-borne diseases. As the physician in charge of Puerto Vallarta's Blood Bank, I saw dozens of local tropical disease-related issues, mostly dengue fever and, in some cases, chagas or chikungunya. One day, I detected abnormal issues in people who were interested in donating their blood. Further study led me to discover other blood-borne diseases that existed locally, ultimately guiding me to further screen and more comprehensively analyze blood received at blood drives. In some cases, I found small circle-like lesions encrusted in red blood cells, observable by microscope. This was later confirmed by a pathologist to be Babesia. As I descended the deepening rabbit hole, I found myself learning about an array of infections co-existing with Babesia; the most abundant of these being reported worldwide was Lyme though I found it to be very different locally.

Mexico has also been dealing with the complicated TBD, rickettsia, for quite some time. Rickettsia is a general blanket description for bacterial infections that cause a series of symptoms related to tick bite. It was first reported as early as 1896, initially emerging from the Idaho Valley in the US. It wasn't until 1940 when it emerged in human hosts reported in the region of Mexico that shares a border with Arizona. Since then, it has been proliferating throughout our country, making it the number-one TBD of our region. It has infected as many as 10 million Mexicans so far versus the almost two million confirmed cases of *Borrelia burgdorferi*. Statistically and currently, the most prevalent TBD pathogens are *Rickettsia rickettssi, Rickettsia typhi* and *Ehrlichia canis*.[175]

Taking a little personal detour before focusing back on Lyme,

Puerto Vallarta, as a destination, is quite exquisite to visit. It is a Mexican beach resort city situated on the Pacific Ocean. It is the city where I currently reside and have my medical practice, and where I wage an active war against this TBD epidemic. 'PV', or simply 'Vallarta', is the second largest urban center in the state of Guadalajara after the Guadalajara Metropolitan Area. The municipality has an area of 1300.7 square kilometers (502.19 square miles) with population centers outside of the city extending from Boca de Tomatlan to the Nayarit border (the Ameca River).

With this being said, Puerto Vallarta is not considered an endemic region for Lyme per se; however, it does attract around four million visitors a year from every part of the world, including highly endemic Lyme regions of the US and Europe. There are overall 40 million international tourists who visit Mexico in general, making it the eighth most popular destination in the world in 2017. Let's not ignore the billions of birds, mammals and lizards that could be potential carriers of vector-borne infections which are excluded from databases and that have no registry of admission or examination. This means that we are possibly more vulnerable to tick- borne diseases than we actually know. However, if truth be told, the cases reported locally are few in numbers, including among tourists visiting PV via cruise ship or taking a horseriding trip, later reporting a diagnosis of Lyme disease after their departure. These reported cases are as few as a handful a month and even just a couple during some months, not nearly as close in number as other areas of the country where thousands of cases have been reported throughout the years, the first patients diagnosed in Mexico being in 1991 in the region of Baja California and Tamaulipas, reportedly suffering from debilitating symptoms and displaying a rash. We also have to take into consideration the fact that several cases fall under the category of 'undiagnosed or misdiagnosed', and do not figure in these reports, most of which most likely go untreated. Unfortunately, the absence of these reported cases creates a possible future issue that contributes to the continuous spread of this frustrating disease.

Chapter 22

Diagnosis

As is in other places around the world, when it comes to diagnosing a tick-borne disease, there are great challenges to obtaining a sensitive and specific test result that concurs with the clinical diagnosis. We have top researchers developing new technologies and techniques to address this issue, most of whom are located in Mexico City and the northern states bordering the US. I have collaborated with medical researchers who I consider the top experts in the field, and have seen false negatives and positives even in the best conditions.

Unfortunately, these occurrences cause testing to be viewed as unreliable – vulnerable to either possible contamination or not being sufficiently sensitive/precise, leading to a false negative result when it could in fact be positive.

Furthermore, as an additional disadvantage, the majority of Mexican physicians are not 'Lyme literate', and will use the generic lab testing with approximately 70 per cent accuracy instead of using the more specialized testing available. According to the ILADS 2017 Health Provider Directory, I am the only member of ILADS (International Lyme and Associated Disease Society) from Mexico, although this year's meeting did see a few other compatriots looking into becoming members themselves. However, though there are very few 'Lyme-literate' Mexican physicians, and even fewer of those who are up to date with international standards, this does not necessarily reflect widespread unfamiliarity with the disease. Mexican people can be highly resourceful: healthcare providers who are interested in learning can receive the latest information via local Lyme meetings, forums and summits throughout the country. These gatherings are usually organized by associations, mainly comprised of patients and their families as well as their doctors.

Consequently, as in other places around the world, we learn from our patients, and they become an important element in the Lyme landscape. Thus, most Lyme awareness and education in Mexico is promoted by groups of people who are in some way related or connected to a patient. In these meetings, doctors and healthcare providers talk about their experiences, what alternatives they've used, protocols, published and pending studies and other useful topics for the Lyme community. If I would venture to compare the meetings in Mexico with those on similar topics I've attended in other parts of the world, I could safely conclude: 'Everyone ignores something and also everyone knows something.'

Research and statistics

Below are most of the published studies relating to Lyme and human rickettsiosis in Mexico. Interestingly it is not a long list for a dilemma that has been with us for quite some time. This begs the question, 'Are the number of cases reported correct?' Probably not.

- 1991 – The first cases were confirmed in the regions of Yucatan, Baja California, Tamaulipas, Mexico City, Sinaloa and Monterrey.[176]
- 1999 – The Nations Epidemiology report detected a prevalence of 1.1 per cent of *B. burgdorferi* in the general population.[177]
- 2003 – More than 3 per cent of deer in the northern part of Mexico were found to have *B. burgdorferi*.[178]
- 2003 – The prevalence of *B. burgdorferi* infection in people in the Northeast region was found to be 6.2 per cent and in Mexico City 3.4 per cent.[179]
- 2007 – The first cases of Lyme disease are reported with abnormal characteristics, such as neurological, cutaneous (skin) and extra articular (joint) symptoms.[180]
- 2010 – In the first large study, 72 pediatric cases were evaluated for symptom detection and serology tests.[181]

Chapter 22

The politics

Lyme disease is a political and controversial medical topic throughout Mexico, much as it is throughout most of the civilized nations of the world. Mexican medical associations still take their cues from the official pronouncements of the powerful US medical organizations, the CDC and the IDSA among them. However, the medical community is bitterly divided, misinformed and purposefully misled by the professional organizations that govern standard medical protocols.

For whatever reason, the powerful medical interests are stubbornly resistant to the concept of 'chronic Lyme disease' or 'post-treatment Lyme disease'. They hedge their bets that all Lyme disease cases fall within a neat little catchall that will definitely be cured within 10 to 30 days with a standard course of antibiotics. Any other outcome is not Lyme disease. Any subsequent patient complaints after this course of treatment, or a recurrence after a period of time, calls for a psychiatric evaluation. The patient is labeled as crazy or depressed for complaining about 'psychosomatic' symptoms.

The current Mexican guidelines, *Guias de Practica Clinica* (GPC), provided by the Federal Department of Health (our equivalent to the US CDC) for the treatment of Lyme disease infections, have not been revised since 2012; thus, the version in current use has not taken into account any of the subsequent developments and research into the disease.[182] Lyme, or what is more generally described as 'spirochete infection', as well as rickettsia, are found in the section categorized as 'infectious exanthemas of infancy', along with CMV (cytomegalovirus), EBV (Epstein Barr virus) and measles. (You can also find a brief description in the section for acute myocarditis and optical neuritis). Inside the infections chapter, Lyme is referred to strictly as a bacterial infection caused by *Borrelia burgdorferi sensu lato*, which is transmitted only by the Ixodes tick. Other strains of Borrelia are not mentioned and there is a separate chapter for rickettsial infections in the typhus section.

Lyme, as per the Mexican guidelines, is defined as a multi-system disease that involves primarily the skin, central nervous system, heart and joints. In addition, it is sub-categorized as 'early localized with an EM rash', 'early disseminated' or 'chronic'. Lastly, one of the most crucial points made in the Guide is that there are no reliable, standardized cultures available, and that the interpretation of other tests (i.e. serology) is oftentimes difficult and unreliable. Treatment is recommended to be done at the doctor's discretion by administering oral doxycycline for seven to 21 days – not more.

As I mentioned before, because the 2012 guidelines have not taken into account subsequent developments, as in the US, giant gaps in diagnosis, treatment and overall medical education/knowledge are apparent. There are, however, other guidelines proposed by respected Mexican medical institutions and health associations involved in TBD that have recommended other means of diagnosis, warning health providers about false negative testing as well as failed cases treated by short courses of antibiotics.

Unfortunately, doctors who follow the GPC guidelines may see higher percentages of false negative cases and are consequently doomed to fail in their treatment plans. Sadly, this adherence to faulty guidelines may subject their patients to unnecessary or flawed treatment plans based on erroneous diagnoses. In some cases, patients are deemed either severely mentally ill or completely healthy when that is certainly not the case. In my opinion, there are a number of mental health facilities filled with undiagnosed Lyme patients as well as tens of thousands of patients hopelessly roaming hospitals and doctors' offices on a daily basis without knowing the actual cause of their long list of puzzling symptoms.

Summary

Most Mexican healthcare providers share the belief that Lyme disease is a simple, self-limiting problem that is easy to treat. However, since there is no current consensus on the matter, we are not yet forced to follow a specific, conventional course of action with unresponsive cases. Thus, here in Mexico, there is some room for experimentation and freedom for physicians to be creative without being harassed, persecuted, expelled, disbarred or discredited, as many healthcare providers have been in other countries. That is the political climate here for now at least.

In terms of progress, Mexico currently enjoys a vibrant, evolving, innovative and collaborative medical research sector with many opportunities that are often encouraged and supported by government programs. Some of these government programs even fund all necessary lab equipment and research materials along with providing cash prizes for the development of new methods in science, technology and overall medical advancement to treat various local, and international, pressing concerns. Therefore, regardless of some negative and unrelated issues that we experienced during this past presidential term of Enrique Pena Nieto, we have also seen successful changes for which to be very thankful.

A specific instance of these changes was the President's decision to improve the country's underdeveloped technology and science departments, financing research and development projects for the greater good, ultimately enhancing his reputation as well as that of Mexico. These benefits include government created and funded programs, subsidies, grants and opportunities, many in the medical field. This has afforded us a unique opportunity to work with new therapies and perform experimental treatments as long as:

1. there is sufficient clinical evidence to support them
2. the person administering them has a research degree and training
3. all the necessary tools and facilities have valid permits.

Therefore, many Mexican doctors are allowed to perform relatively experimental, alternative therapies as long as they have the requisite certificate to prove that they are trained in doing so and that they comply with the above requirements. Some treatments, such as the ones we utilize with some of our Lyme and co-infection patients (such as administering plasmapheresis or blood transfusions), require more rigorous prerequisites, yet they are still more readily available in Mexico than in other countries. For example, we are able to take and administer any number of blood components to and from anyone without any restrictions, given that it is deemed necessary and appropriate for the patient.

In conclusion, although there are many shortcomings when it comes to public understanding of tick-borne disease in Mexico, by using research methods, there is a world of opportunity for those who are literate in Lyme and co-infections seeking alternatives that can be practiced in the comfort of private hospitals and clinics. I, personally, have seen joyless faces suddenly light up with hope and exhilaration when someone tells them that they are not crazy, that they do have Lyme disease, that they have been misdiagnosed and that there are steps that can be taken to get them better. These are generally my personal favorite consultations and fill me with satisfaction regarding what we are able to do for these patients.

Chapter 23

Addressing the global human rights violations of Lyme patients and their human rights defenders

Jenna Luché-Thayer

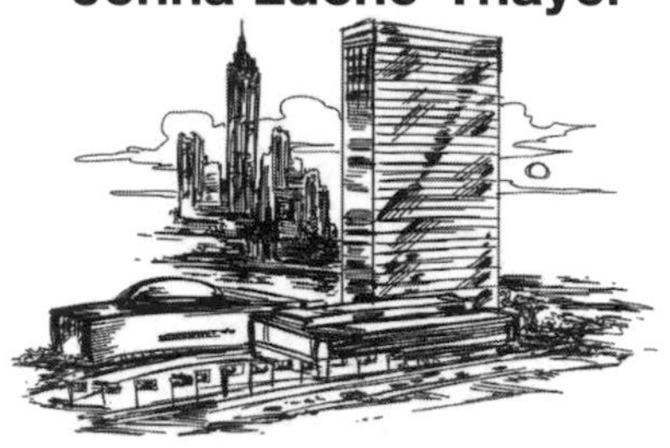

'ACCESSIBILITY: Health facilities, goods, and services have to be accessible
(physically accessible, affordable, and supported by accessible information) to everyone
within the jurisdiction of the State party without discrimination.'
WHO principles

My name is Jenna Luché-Thayer and I am a former Senior Adviser to the United Nations (UN) and US Government and a recognized expert on government transparency, accountability and human rights. My global career has spanned 33 years and 42 countries, and it is my love of nature and professional experience that brought me into Lyme advocacy.

I suffered from systemic Lyme infection for at least 17 years before being correctly diagnosed. Nearly all of my international work with rural farming communities and recreational activities exposed me to ticks. Prior to my Lyme diagnosis, my misdiagnoses included fibromyalgia, depression, irritable bowel syndrome, lupus, chronic fatigue syndrome, multiple sclerosis and two additional autoimmune diseases. Fortunately, my scientific training and self-awareness helped me to recognize these diagnoses did not match my overall constellation of symptoms so I did not take the drugs prescribed for these illnesses, many of which are immunosuppressive.

The Lyme diagnosis, however, did match my health history and so I underwent the long-term antimicrobial treatment that has been vetted through the clinical practice guidelines that have met the internationally accepted standards set by the Institute of Medicine in 2011.

Following these extended antimicrobial treatments, my infection went into remission and I regained my energy and health.

During my period of antimicrobial treatment, I became very well informed regarding certain political and economic factors surrounding the global Lyme epidemic. I was shocked to find the science and medical practices regarding Lyme that were promoted by the CDC, and health authorities in other countries, had little to do with the realities of the disease or helping Lyme patients. I found these policies and practices promoted significant human rights violations and had everything to do with obvious conflicts of interest, such as collusion between State Actors, certain private medical societies and insurers.

As an advocate for gender equality, I had been involved in the political action to overturn the CDC's denial that heterosexual women were contracting HIV / AIDS. I was well aware the CDC had contrived a narrow case definition for the disease that for over 14 years excluded the symptoms HIV-positive women manifested … and this obstructed medical care for women living with HIV. This sexist practice was a politically motivated decision to deny the epidemic.

I have provided expert testimony to governments in numerous countries and the United Nations; these include cases featuring corruption and State-sponsored discrimination and human rights violations. My expertise includes the political empowerment of marginalized groups and corporate social responsibility. I have worked with governments, the UN, non-profits and the corporate world and have authored over 75 publications. I have received international awards for my advocacy on behalf of marginalized populations, including the International Woman's Day Award for Exemplary Dedication and Contributions to Improving the Political and Legal Status of Women (US Government), and built the Highest Ranking Technical Area in Accomplishment, Innovation and Comparative Advantage for United Nations Capital Development Fund, the UN agency established to politically engage and bring services to the most marginalized in the world, and most recently the ILADS Power of Lyme Award 2017.

As a global expert in transparency and accountability, I had become increasingly aware of how the pharmaceutical and health insurance industries were corrupting healthcare systems across the globe.

However, when I assessed the circumstances surrounding the Lyme epidemic, I found these corrupting influences had hit a new order of magnitude and become embedded into healthcare systems across many nations and both the governmental and intergovernmental bodies responsible for public health. It appeared to me none of these key institutions had made consistent or concerted efforts to correct these threats to the many millions of persons across the globe at risk of exposure to the Lyme-borreliosis infection. I was not alone in my views and assessments and found there were many professionals across the globe who shared these concerns and were willing to take action to address the situation.

In 2016, I had a conversation with Dr Ken Liegner regarding the poorly articulated codes for Lyme borreliosis (LB); they lacked most of the complications from LB, including those that are life-threatening, such as congenital Lyme and dementia from Lyme. With Dr Liegner's help, I founded the all-voluntary Ad Hoc Committee for Health Equity in ICD11 Borreliosis Codes (Ad Hoc Committee). The Ad Hoc Committee is part of the global borreliosis community that includes non-governmental organizations, scientists, medical professionals, patient groups, government officials and elected officials. The Ad Hoc Committee was initially formed to update WHO's International Classification of Disease (ICD) codes, version 10, for LB and demonstrate how the outdated codes are contributing to human rights violations and medical marginalization.

The Ad Hoc Committee's members represent highly skilled professionals from North and South America, the Asia Pacific region, Africa, and Eastern, Western and Northern Europe. Many members are scientific and medical experts and have worked on borreliosis for two or three decades, and among them have many hundreds of peer-reviewed publications and studies. They serve as leaders, clinicians and professors across numerous well-respected academic and research centers. Many members consult regularly to the WHO and governments on the development of health systems, surveillance practices, patient-centered care, aging, zoonosis, climate change and other specialized areas. Other members are experts in law, medical fraud, institutional reform, citizen mobilization, and capacity building.

The ICD10 codes for LB generally follow the narrow case definition of the disease, which is intended for many purposes, including surveillance. The specific ICD10 code for Lyme is A69.2 and includes meningitis due to LB and some neurological disorders, and arthritis due to LB. Lyme carditis, a complication of LB 'officially recognized' by health authorities, is not even noted in these codes.

Like LB, syphilis is also a spirochetal infection and its complications are similar to those of LB. In contrast, the WHO allocates five times more codes to syphilis than to Lyme; with syphilis, almost every manifestation is listed under its syphilis-specific code, whereas the Lyme codes are missing many manifestations of the condition that are described in peer-reviewed publications, many of which can be fatal.

ICD10 codes include rare and quirky conditions, such as

'W61.62XD Struck by duck', 'W55.1 Bitten by a cow', 'V91.07 Burn due to water skis on fire', 'V95.40 Unspecified spacecraft accident injuring occupant' and 'R46.1 Bizarre personal appearance'.

The attention to coding for syphilis and 'spacecraft injury' in contrast to the lack of code articulation for the many manifestations of LB is one indicator of the powerful financial and political interests driving the human suffering of the Lyme epidemic.

Another indicator is the 'evidence-based science' and uniform code logic used to develop the ICD codes. In the case of LB, WHO appears to have a standing practice of ignoring hundreds of peer-reviewed publications on LB and the thousands of LB patient testimonials on record across the parliaments and congresses of their member states. The outdated and insufficient ICD10 LB codes have led to decades of suppressed numbers in surveillance data and the retention of public health policies that appear uncaring and are ineffective and harmful.

In most countries, the electronic medical information systems, which are embedded with these codes, restrict how Lyme disease is recorded and reported. As noted, there are no codes for many serious and life-threatening LB manifestations. When a condition found in a certain illness does not match a code, the electronic system defaults to the 'unspecified illness' category and this usually results in an 'experimental treatment' for an 'unspecified illness' or 'unspecified condition'. When clinical decision support software is utilized to identify any one of the LB manifestations missing from the codes, the software will recommend non-specific 'experimental treatment' for 'unspecified illness' or 'unspecified condition'. Therefore, many LB patients will find their treatments are not covered or reimbursed and they may be obstructed from any access to medical care for their biological illness. Creating systems that obstruct access to care or have coverage practices that exclude subsets of patients within a patient group, is in opposition to health human rights.

At the core of this systemic violation of the human rights of Lyme and relapsing fever borreliosis patients are the WHO's

ICD codes. The ICD codes are created in a collaborative process engaging the member states, WHO and experts identified for various working groups on specific topics, such as infectious diseases. It is likely that within this labyrinth of collaborative processes that the corrupted financial and political influences shape the outcomes.

Despite LB being recognized as a disease of consequence for decades, WHO has yet to sponsor a meeting with LB patients suffering from persistent LB infection, or Lyme complicated by co-infections, or medical experts who have successfully treated the patients who suffer with the persistent and complicated forms of the disease. Again, the marginalization of this patient group and their human rights defenders stands in sharp contrast to how WHO routinely engages with patients and their medical specialists from *other diseases of consequence*.

The Ad Hoc Committee's report, *Updating ICD11 Borreliosis Diagnostic Codes*, was accepted by WHO prior to the 30 March 2017 deadline for code revisions. Also, as per WHO's required rules and process for ICD revisions, each recommendation from the report was entered onto the WHO ICD Beta Platform. The Ad Hoc Committee ensured that no less than three peer-reviewed publications supported each and every entry we made.

According to the WHO stated procedure, any recommendations to the ICD11 Beta Platform that are rejected would be preceded by a 'digital conversation' between WHO and the person who entered the recommendation onto the Platform. Initially most of the Ad Hoc Committee's Beta Platform recommendations were rejected with no conversation or reason given (with the exception of one recommendation that noted 'this condition was under discussion' – paraphrased). This exceptional behavior by the WHO for the LB recommendations is very striking given the many hundreds of conversations registered across the Beta Platform for other diseases and medical conditions, many of which resulted in accepting the related recommendation.

The *Updating ICD11 Borreliosis Diagnostic Codes* report was also submitted to Dr Dainius Pūras, the United Nations Human Rights Council's Special Rapporteur for the right of everyone to enjoy the highest attainable standard of physical and mental health.

Dr Pūras held a meeting with the Ad Hoc Committee in Geneva on 7 June 2017.

He accepted all the Ad Hoc Committee's documentation, including reports, books and videos, PowerPoint and verbal testimony and outlined how he could support this effort within the framework of his mandate. The topics included how medical practitioners had collectively and effectively treated tens of thousands of patients with persistent and complicated LB with clinical practice guidelines that have met internationally accepted standards and that there are accredited educational programs on how to implement such therapies. The main report included hundreds of peer-reviewed studies – written by nationally and internationally recognized scientists and medical researchers from across the globe – describing:

> *Congenital Lyme disease, persistent infection, Borrelial lymphocytoma, Granuloma annulare, morphea, localized scleroderma, lichen sclerosis and atrophicus, Lyme meningitis, Lyme nephritis, Lyme hepatitis, Lyme myositis, Lyme aortic aneurysm, coronary artery aneurysm, late Lyme endocarditis, Lyme carditis, late Lyme neuritis or neuropathy, meningovascular and neuro borreliosis – with cerebral infarcts, intracranial aneurysm, Lyme parkinsonism, late Lyme meningoencephalitis or meningomyelo-encephalitis, atrophic form of Lyme meningoencephalitis with dementia and subacute pre-senile dementia, neuropsychiatric manifestations, late Lyme disease of liver and other viscera, late Lyme disease of kidney and ureter, late Lyme disease of bronchus and lung, and seronegative and latent Lyme disease, unspecified.*

Altogether, these documents and testimony established the scientific facts that patients with persistent Lyme and Lyme and co-infections require medical care for biological illness. The record also showed many human rights violations against the Lyme patient group and their human rights defenders. These included how medical practitioners who treat this patient group are routinely defamed, falsely accused of wrongdoing, capriciously penalized, and threatened with loss of license and livelihood. This led to the Ad Hoc Committee meeting with the Special Rapporteur, Michel Forst, who is responsible for the situation of human rights defenders.

The ICD10 codes are linked to policies recommending practices that:

- for many patients, prevent proper diagnosis and obstruct access to treatment options that meet internationally accepted standards
- promote discrimination based on illness manifestations
- misapply a psychosomatic diagnosis that is then used to obstruct medical care for biological illness
- obstruct treatments based on illness manifestations
- promote discrimination based on financial status
- support attacks on human rights defenders – including medical practitioners, scientists and researchers who act on behalf of this vulnerable patient group
- restrict information regarding treatment options that meet internationally accepted standards
- routinely exclude key stakeholders – such as medical practitioners, researchers, patients and caretakers who are concerned with persistent and complicated cases of LB – from decision-making venues, making these stakeholders invisible to policy makers, economists and other practitioners and researchers
- forcibly remove sick children receiving treatments that meet internationally accepted standards from their parents – and there are many cases where such parents have been falsely accused of poisoning their children (Munchausen's syndrome by proxy)

- in some alarming cases, encourage euthanasia over treatments that meet internationally accepted standards.

One example is the exposure of the role of the government of Denmark in human rights abuse. For years, the government of Denmark hid a foundational conflict of interest of one academic who advised them on the recommended ELISA serology tests and the fact that he is a patent owner for that test in Denmark. There is increasing evidence the government of Denmark has suppressed the public knowledge of the epidemic because their national health system cannot afford to address the epidemic. In fact, the government owned the TV2 network that was used to produce a propaganda documentary that stigmatized Lyme patients as hypochondriacs and fools and attacked German laboratories that used a diagnostic technology that had been approved and implemented in many nations and across scientific institutions. including academic centers of research.

There are many more examples including corrupt health insurance companies who collude with a stable of expert witnesses to deny coverage and treatment, alliances between academics and State Actors who ensured that millions in grant monies would bolster national health policies that ignored this patient group, or stigmatized them as hypochondriacs and therefore unable to access medical care or disability support, and the ravening pharmaceutical companies who profited greatly by having undiagnosed, untreated and undertreated Lyme patients purchase expensive and dangerous symptom-modifying drugs for the remainder of their lives ... or until their money runs out, whichever comes first.

These models of corruption have been identified by many scholars and there are ethical members of government and private enterprises trying to remove this unsustainable rot. On January 30 2018 the companies Amazon, Berkshire Hathaway, and JPMorgan Chase announced a partnership to cut health costs and improve services for over one million employees by creating an independent operation that would be 'free from profit-making incentives'. The US stock market lost hundreds of points following this announcement, another indication of just how deep this corruption runs.

The widespread discrimination experienced by Lyme patients has been systemic and institutionalized across ICD codes, national health policies, healthcare and insurance systems. Altogether, these factors have led to gross human rights violations that are on record with the United Nations Human Rights Council's Special Rapporteur for the right of everyone to enjoy the highest attainable standard of physical and mental health. This record will continue to grow and be widely disseminated until few politicians and policymakers can plead ignorance of the role of profit-making incentives and politics in the inhumane and degrading treatment of Lyme patients.

Correcting the codes for Lyme is a very manageable task that has worldwide impacts. These impacts include improving the lives of patients who need to access treatment options, reducing the length of time between clinical diagnosis and treatment, and thereby reducing the risk of disability and death for the many millions of people across the globe who are exposed to Lyme borreliosis. This reasonably simple task will only be undertaken when there are sufficient numbers of strong, courageous and ethical people willing to challenge and fight back against the ugly politics of this pandemic.

The Ad Hoc Committee received historic news on June 18 2018 when the draft ICD11 was released. For the first time in over 25 years, the LB codes had been significantly increased, by almost 400 per cent, and included life-threatening complications. WHO and ICD11, however, do not acknowledge post-treatment Lyme disease syndrome (PTLDS).

PTLDS was fabricated by the IDSA and 'officially introduced' in the 2006 IDSA Guidelines for LB. Since its introduction by the IDSA and its dissemination by the IDSA, the CDC and others, PTLDS has caused great global harm to Lyme patients. Both governmental and private insurers have abused the term 'post treatment' to deny care and coverage of LB care. The diagnosis of PTLDS usually results in palliative care for LB patients, even when they are children at the start of life.

In December 2018, WHO's acknowledgement of LB was then seriously undermined when, in a completely non-transparent process, the code for congenital LB disappeared from ICD11. WHO's stated reasons for removing this code do not answer the questions I and others have posed to WHO. I have the original communications from by a member of the WHO ICD11 Medical and Scientific Committee stating the removal of the code for congenital Lyme borreliosis came at the request of the Public Health Agency of Canada.

How many millions of children across the globe will be disabled or die because of this unilateral action by certain officials in the Public Health Agency of Canada?

This unilateral action by the Public Health Agency of Canada will result in millions of children across the globe becoming disabled and dying from this disease. In this case, WHO has failed to follow its own rules for transparency and will also be responsible for this unnecessary suffering and death.

In fact, the new code for congenital LB should inspire nations to change their health policies whereby women who are pregnant or planning to become pregnant are routinely screened for LB.

The Ad Hoc Committee for Health Equity in ICD11 Borreliosis Codes is part of an emerging global movement dedicated to overturning the suppression of science and medical knowledge regarding persistent and complicated LB and the corruption driving the related horrific human rights abuses. These efforts are becoming better coordinated, the resulting information is being documented and put on record with key institutions, and more government officials and politicians are becoming aware of the corruption and unconscionable motives behind these policies and practices. The failures in addressing the Lyme epidemic have been gaining widespread acknowledgment. On November 15 2018, the European Parliament unanimously endorsed a resolution for Lyme stating:

> *Lyme borreliosis is the most common zoonotic disease in Europe… infected ticks and the disease seem to be expanding geographically … a bite by an infected tick and the symptoms of Lyme disease can go unnoticed or even in some cases be asymptomatic, which can sometimes lead to severe complications and permanent damage similar to that of a chronic disease, in particular when the patient is not promptly diagnosed.*
>
> *Lyme disease is still underdiagnosed, in particular because of the difficulties encountered in the detection of symptoms and the absence of appropriate diagnostic tests; many patients are neither promptly diagnosed nor have access to suitable treatment; more reliable early diagnosis of Lyme disease will significantly reduce the number of later-stage cases, thus improving quality of life for patients; it will also reduce the financial burden of the disease…*
>
> *The International Lyme and Associated Diseases Society treatment practice guidelines differ from those of Infectious Diseases Society of America and these differences between the two approaches to the disease also have an impact on treatment practices in the EU:*
>
> *'The medical profession often follows outdated recommendations on Lyme disease that do not take sufficient account of research developments ... health professionals have been sounding the alarm about this health issue for nearly a decade, as have patients' associations and whistle-blowers …'*

There are no separate codes in the International Classification of Diseases (ICD) for early and advanced stages of Lyme disease and no unique ICD codes for the different symptoms of advanced stage Lyme disease; this calls for ICD code separation between early-stage and late-stage Lyme disease; this calls also for individual ICD codes for the different late-stage Lyme disease symptoms.'

As part of my efforts to educate the public why the proper representation of LB in the ICD codes may address the related corruption and human rights abuse, I authored *Lyme, How Medical Codes Mortally Wound Corruption and Scientific Fraud,* illustrated by David Skidmore. This has reached a global readership and is currently being translated into Swedish, French, Spanish and German. More details regarding LB-related corruption and human rights violations may be found in the two reports by the Ad Hoc Committee that were submitted to the Special Rapporteurs and WHO. The reports are *The Situation of Human Rights Defenders of Lyme and Relapsing Fever Borreliosis Patients* (Edition One, March 6, 2018) and *Updating ICD11 Borreliosis Diagnostic Codes* (Edition One, March 29, 2017).*

* Lyme and the Ad Hoc Committee's two reports to the UN may be purchased from Amazon; Lyme is found under 'true crime' and 'organized crime'.

Part Five

Patient healing

The following section features writing from my former patient, author and Lyme advocate, Allie Cashel. Allie has been lost in the Lyme maze herself, but thankfully, has found her way out. We leave you with her story.

Chapter 24

Suffering the Silence Journey through the Lyme labyrinth

Allie Cashel

I can't remember the waiting room or the office, but I do remember the chair. The legs and arms were thick plastic made to look like wood, with a hard plastic cushion on the seat made to look like fabric. I sat in that chair for more than an hour, trying to trick my brain into accepting the illusion of comfort while I shifted my weight around and waited.

It was 2008. My mother and I were meeting with a new doctor that day – one of the best in the business of pediatric infectious disease. As a 17-year-old, I was still a minor and not in any state to handle my own appointments. I was lost in an onslaught of neurological symptoms that left my family desperate for answers. In just a few months, I had gone from a high functioning high school student to a child who was sleeping upwards of 18 hours a day, who was struggling to speak and read, who could not safely drive a car. The symptoms had come on hard and fast, and they were unlike anything we had ever seen before.

The trouble was, we had seen lots of symptoms and doctors' offices in the years leading up to the fall of 2008. I had first been diagnosed with Lyme disease 10 years earlier, in 1998. The initial diagnosis was uncomplicated. I had a tick bite, a bullseye rash, a fever, a positive blood test. Everything a mainstream doctor needs to make a clean, early-stage diagnosis, I had. I was prescribed a short course of antibiotics to treat the infection and assumed I was cured. I went back to my life playing in the grass and climbing trees and forgot about Lyme and tick-borne disease for as long as I could.

But when I started to go through puberty around 12 years old, I noticed strange symptoms that other kids my age were not experiencing. By the end of middle school, those symptoms were impossible to ignore. I was in constant joint and muscle pain, sometimes so bad that I struggled to walk. My sensitivity to light and sound shaped every moment of the day and the tremors in my arms and legs were both embarrassing and exhausting.

When a local doctor approached my parents to ask if I had ever been diagnosed with Lyme disease, the question didn't come as much of a surprise. I grew up in Westchester County, just about an hour north of New York City and one of the most endemic areas for Lyme in the US. Though I had been treated and diagnosed before, it wasn't hard to imagine that I could have been re-infected without knowing it. All of my symptoms still fell cleanly into a textbook Lyme case and the blood work continued to come back positive.

At the time of that second diagnosis, my family and I did not know that we were stepping into a dark forest, a confusing and controversial world where every doctor we spoke to had different answers and different recommendations, and where we struggled to find treatments that would keep symptoms at bay for longer than a few months. The 'Lyme maze', as Dr Raxlen has so aptly named it, was a place we realized we were in only once we had got deep into it. No one warned us of the complexity of this maze, of the toll it would take on our family and on my body. No one gave us a flashlight to illuminate the darkest corners. It was only once we were stuck inside that we realized how hard it would be to escape.

Consistent guidance or advice has always been hard to come by in the Lyme world. I can't tell you how hungry I was to hear physicians agree with each other, to find some type of consistent messaging and clarity during the peak of my journey with tick-borne disease. I never had that clarity. Instead, I was presented with two directly conflicting viewpoints while struggling to survive in what felt like two separate worlds. As with the cases Dr Raxlen has described earlier in this book, I hope that my story will provide some insight into tactics and practices that will help those lost in the Lyme maze find their way out again.

I first started working with Dr Raxlen at a pivotal moment in my tick-borne disease treatment. I was re-diagnosed with Lyme disease by our local physician and went through a series of oral medications without seeing much improvement. Ultimately, the local doctor recommended we increase the strength of my treatment and prescribed daily intravenous (IV) antibiotic therapy. During my freshman year of high school, I would spend over an hour at her office every day before school, sitting hooked up to an IV line, fluids slowly making their way through my bloodstream. This was as emotionally draining as it was physically exhausting, and though my symptoms improved, they didn't clear. After more than six months without improvement and without additional suggestions from the doctor, my family and I left the clinic in search of new help.

My father had also been struggling with tick-borne disease quite seriously for some time. He had seen success with Dr Raxlen at his office in Greenwich, so just before my sophomore year in high school we made an appointment at his office. After completing yet another round of tests and oral antibiotic trials, Dr Raxlen started me on a PICC line (peripherally inserted central catheter), and I finished up my longest and most aggressive round of antibiotic treatment with him that year.

My junior year of high school, the year that followed, was by far the healthiest that I could remember. I was able to go off of antibiotics and started working with a naturopathic doctor in Connecticut to build my body back up after all that treatment. He started addressing the candida issues and the massive nutrient deficiencies I had in my body. I was still in and out of his office for treatment all the time, but I felt healthier than I had ever been. And, perhaps most importantly, I felt like I had my life back. I was thriving academically and socially, and once again it seemed like Lyme was behind me.

I could feel myself coming out of my own shell. As a younger person, I had always been quite shy, but it was hard to know whether or not that was due to my experience with illness. I had missed weeks of school every year, and even on the days that I was there, I had regularly missed classes for doctors' appointments and treatments. I had rarely told classmates about Lyme. Only my closest friends knew what was going on day to day, and even they didn't know the extent of my challenge with the disease.

I was afraid that people would think I was weak and chose not to let anyone look behind the curtain at the struggles of day-to-day life. So when that struggle started to fade into the background, I felt, for the first time since I had been a little girl, like I was able to be myself.

Then, the summer before my senior year of high school, my father landed a job in Boston, and my family needed to relocate. As I was finally feeling healthy and starting to get into the swing of things at school, my parents and I decided it would be best for me to stay in New York and finish school there. I'd live with a family friend in our house until it sold and would commute back and forth to see my parents whenever I could.

That summer, all of my tick-borne disease symptoms slowly started to make their way back into my life. Stress can be a powerful trigger, but at the time I didn't know the effect it could have on my body. Within just a few weeks of starting school that fall, I fell into my first major neurological flare and was overwhelmed by symptoms I had never experienced before. I was struggling to read and write and getting lost on my way to school or around the building. I was in six car accidents in just six weeks. Something was very wrong.

I have days, maybe even weeks, during that time that I can hardly remember. Memories exist almost like blurry images without sound or texture. But the thing I remember more than anything else is the fear. I had lost all control over my life and all awareness of how I could get it back. The seductive period of health the year before made this fall back into illness even more debilitating.

My parents pulled me out of school and brought me to Boston in an effort to get answers to these new and scary symptoms. We, of course considered tick-borne disease as a possibility, but this was unlike any experience of Lyme or TBD that we had ever known. We were desperate for help, for someone who could explain with a clarity that resonated with our previous experiences and understandings.

This brings me back to that waiting room and plastic chair. My parents had arranged an appointment with one of the best pediatricians in the Boston area. My mother took me to the appointment and I remember we laughed for the first time in ages on the way there. In our minds, this doctor was a true expert, someone who held all the information and who could shine a light on our darkness.

When we arrived at his office he brought my mother into his examination room, leaving me behind to wait. He spent over an hour talking to her about my medical history and my current symptom presentation. At no point did he conduct a physical examination, or ask me personally to describe how I was feeling. At the end of his conversation with my mom, he brought me into his office and told me that it was physically impossible that my symptoms were related to Lyme or TBD, but instead told me I was regressing to a stage of infancy in response to my parents' move. Effectively, I was having a mental breakdown. It was 'all in my head'.

This dismissal of my symptoms as all in my head created a schism in my family's and my own perception of this disease. Some part of me intrinsically believed he was wrong, but I also believed that doctors knew more than me. Who was I to say that this man was wrong? The doubt was overpowering. My family experienced that same dualism, split between believing that

Lyme was real or that it was not. The hurt and resentment that came from being ignored on both sides was incredibly damaging to our dynamic. Trust was broken, and that is so hard to repair.

When the test results finally came back, I found out I was still dealing with Lyme and also with Babesia, Bartonella and Ehrlichia. And once I had got back to aggressively treating the TBD, I was able to start to see a light at the end of the tunnel again.

It's remarkable to think back on how little information was made available to us in the early days of my Lyme treatment and ultimately in the later years, as I faced a battle with the neurological effects of tick-borne disease. Conversations with physicians, and sometimes even test results, would directly contradict each other just days apart. I had such a limited understanding of what was happening around me that close friends and family members were left in the dark about the details of my experience. It was my parents, my doctors, and me who had to fight our way through the No Man's Land and back to safety again, a path fraught with bumps and wrong turns along the way.

Through my work on this book, and on *Suffering the Silence: Chronic Lyme Disease in an Age of Denial,* I've come to learn that my experience in No Man's Land is not unique. Patients around the world who face Lyme diagnosis and treatment experience the same feelings of loss and confusion that I did. I personally know at least 10 people right now who are struggling to identify the root cause of their illness, who are being passed from physician to physician, who may suspect TBD but who have the idea quickly dismissed by their specialists.

Unlike many of those individuals, and unlike many of the patients' stories presented throughout this book, my case is actually a fairly simple one. I did not see hundreds of doctors in my quest to find answers. I had access to Dr Raxlen and other 'Lyme-literate' doctors (LLMDs), quite early in my journey through TBD. Instead of asking whether or not I had Lyme disease, the question was whether or not I believed Lyme disease was real. Even after what became years of treatment, was it possible that I was still suffering from the effects of a tick-borne infection? This question about the mere existence of infection, or the root cause of my suffering, is ultimately what shaped my own journey through the Lyme maze, through the No Man's Land that so many patients find themselves in around the world.

So, can tick-borne infection persist in the body despite continued antibiotic intervention? This is a question that elicits strong reactions from doctors on both sides of this polarizing debate. But as a patient, the certainty presented by each side can be incredibly confusing. Who do you trust? Why should you trust the LLMD over the infectious disease specialist at your major urban hospital? How do you make that decision for yourself?

In the aftermath of my experience with Lyme, I grappled with many of these questions. It was only during periods of relative health that was I able to come to find my way towards satisfying answers.

Chapter 25

Lyme as teacher and guide

Allie Cashel

This year marks 11 years since my first major neurological flare and 11 years since I learned firsthand how toxic the Lyme world could be. It is not only the disease itself that is hard to recover from, it's also the trauma of navigating the maze, of deciding who to trust and making sure that your voice is one of the voices you always believe.

Today, I am happy to say that I do consider myself to be in remission. Though I still do deal with symptoms that I believe are related to Lyme and Lyme treatment, I think I have the tick-borne disease under control. Remission is a word that suggests that it will probably come back at some point, and I've come to accept that as a potential reality. My life so far has been a series of healthy times and sick times. I have no reason to believe that won't continue, but I do feel that if/when I get sick again, it won't be as bad as it once was.

I've actually been relatively healthy since 2008. Even when things aren't going as well as they should be, nothing has compared to that level of fear or sickness. As I cycle through phases of sickness and health, the focus of my healing has been more emotional than physical, a thought that was once extremely difficult for me to accept.

I graduated from high school six months after I was told I was suffering from a mental breakdown and started college later that summer. When I went off to college, I wasn't nearly as sick as I had been but I was still symptomatic, juggling rounds of treatment with periods of successfully healthy illusions. Though I was successfully keeping up appearances, I still didn't know how to take care of myself, how to accept the waves of sickness and wellness that continue to shape my experience today.

I needed to work on my relationship with my body. I spent so much time trying to convince doctors that something was physically and not emotionally wrong with me that I fell completely out of touch with my emotional experience of both sickness and health. I refused to accept that this trauma would affect me emotionally or psychologically, and that made it almost impossible to fully heal. The turning point came when I accepted the fact that disease was something I needed to live with. It wasn't something I could just wish away. I felt a shift when I finally decided truly to accept my anger, my disease, and that it was my job to take care of my own body.

No one told me that the healing process takes so much time. Even once the infection has cleared, it can take years to get your body systems back in check, to heal emotionally from the experience and to regulate your immune system. Some may have to manage ebbs and flows of symptoms indefinitely, which requires not only major lifestyle changes but also that the patient takes on a certain level of responsibility. We need to own our own healing to see progress.

I wasn't able to accept this and to take responsibility for my own health until I started work on my book, *Suffering the Silence: Chronic Lyme Disease in the Age of Denial*, as mentioned above. Throughout the research process, I had the privilege of talking to many other people about their experiences with Lyme. In listening to their stories, for the first time I saw validity in my own experience. I was able to accept my anger and my confusion as real, and from that point forward, I was able to start healing.

As I've said, I still am in a pretty constant cycle of health and illness. I go through phases where things are fabulous and then phases where things are not. I know the lifestyle choices and diet changes I need to make to support my body, and sometimes I am better than others at implementing these. I am noticing, though, that the sick periods are getting farther and farther apart and are getting shorter and shorter.

I'm living a very normal life these days. And I attribute so much of that to my ability to accept and ultimately to let go of my grief and anger. In some ways, I think that was holding me back from living the life I wanted to be able to live when I got healthy.

This type of healing is not something anyone talked to me about when I first got sick. Or if they did, I wasn't able to hear it. But it's not the only thing that I attribute to getting my life back.

The top things I attribute to getting my life back are:

- Antibiotics and Western medicine: I am a firm believer that if you have an infection, you need to treat it as aggressively as possible. I attribute a lot of my success to the work I did with Dr Raxlen on treating the infections and keeping them at bay.
- Supplements and dietary support: That being said, I also think that you need to make sure your body is strong enough to handle that treatment. For a long time, I didn't take any supplements, much to my parents' and doctors' chagrin. Once I started down a more holistic path, I was able to do much better.
- Acceptance: I couldn't get better until I learned to accept what this disease did to my sense of self, to my body, and to my relationships. Once I could accept that, it was much easier to let go of some of the grief and focus on moving forward.

There are many who will disagree with me, with Dr Raxlen, with the other physicians who contributed to this book, about how to heal and cure this disease. As has been stated a number of times, this is a controversial landscape and patients often have to choose which narratives or which modes of thinking most resonate with them. In today's day and age, we have the power to arm ourselves with incredible amounts of information, but the trouble is that the doctors, or even the other patients who we choose to present it to, do not always believe the information we collect.

The internet has been a transformative tool for the Lyme community and the chronic illness community as a whole, but there can also be many angry and conflicting perspectives that are broadcast there. It is important to remember that the loudest voices are the ones you will hear, not necessarily the smartest or most empathetic. That being said, there are also so many supportive and kind people who are eager to connect with other Lyme and chronic illness sufferers online. Their experiences can be valuable. Learn from them and from what they have been through in their own Lyme journey.

I would also encourage anyone who finds themselves in the midst of this fight to speak up and tell their stories when they are ready. It is important that we learn from each other, and the experience of staying silent, of not speaking up about the complexity of our experiences with illness, is all too common. It is easy to find yourself stuck in a complex world of isolation, one informed both by actual illness/disease and by the feelings of disdain, stigma and disbelief that surround it.

As Susan Sontag writes in her famous book, *Illness as Metaphor*, 'Illness is the night side of life, a more onerous citizenship. Everyone who is born holds dual citizenship, in the kingdom of the well and in the kingdom of the sick. Although we all prefer to use the good passport, sooner or later each of us is obliged, at least for a spell, to identify ourselves as citizens of that other place.'[183]

This is something I'm unfortunately familiar with. I know the 'night side of life' well, and I know how difficult it can be (especially as a young person) to tell people that I've been there. But I also know how helpful it can be to speak up and to connect with others who have travelled to 'the night side'.

Back on the lighter side of life, I still worry about when I'll have to travel back and deal with my symptoms again. But I am now armed with so many resources, so much information, and so much support, that I truly believe that if I do get sick again, I will know what I need to do to get healthy.

When we go through this awful disease, we don't come out with nothing. We come out knowing ourselves much better than we did going in. I think that is an incredible weapon we can use against illness and even in times of health. I encourage everyone fighting these battles to recognize how far they have come and how much they have learned.

Chapter 26

Beyond the rays of hope – David McClain, spiritual transcendence

Dr Bernard Raxlen

Back in 2004, I was one of the physicians privileged in helping a patient named David McClain. During the later period of his intractable ALS (motor neurone disease) he was able to communicate with the world through the ingenious invention of eye movement computer assisted spelling and speech, laboriously moving his eyes over a TV monitor screen, letter by letter. He was able to spell out words and turn them into computer speech, produce written material, blog share personal thoughts and even write poems.

I asked if I could share my personal thoughts about his remarkable story. Since the time I asked for his permission to include this in my book he has passed away peacefully, surrounded by loved ones in his home in February 2019.

I first met Mr David McClain in July 2004. He was a robust father of three, married to his wife Donna for 25 years. He was employed as a manager in a steel company. His initial symptoms were slurred speech, joint pain (in his hips, shoulders and toes), tired jaw cramping in his throat (he found it difficult to sing) and trouble swallowing. He had received a tick bite two years before he first visited me on his right thigh and a second tick bite one year later. He had seen a number of specialist physicians and had had electrocardiography which proved negative.

On examination, his right eye was able to focus only laterally, and he showed pharyngeal nerve weakness with a deviation of his tongue. His right thumb and first fingers showed weak strength and his overall grip was weak. Other symptoms included testicular pain, lower abdominal pain and an inability to power enough air to blow his nose.

With David's history of tick exposure, and his neurological symptoms following within 24 months, a diagnosis of neuroborreliosis with bulbar involvement was made clinically by myself, and confirmed by Dr Katz, a neurologist in Connecticut familiar with the condition David was exhibiting. He was placed on IV antibiotic therapy and immediately responded in a positive manner. He reported more energy and was able to go to the gym to work out; his breathing had also improved. At night, there was decreased drooling and he was able to blow his nose.

His diploplia (double vision) had disappeared and there was no indication of any more hip pain and minimal joint pain. In addition, there were no more night sweats and there were no problems with cramping. This improvement was reported after eight months of completing IV antibiotic therapy. Mr McClain was feeling well enough to travel again for the steel company and was doing a remarkable 100 push-ups daily.

Fast forward to April 2016.

In spite of what appeared to be a remission after the IV antibiotic therapy, Mr McClain's medical condition took a turn for the worst and in a relatively short time following his improvement in 2005 he went rapidly downhill, going from a wheelchair to being completely bed ridden.

As he has described so poignantly:

I lay motionless for 23 of the 24 hours each day.

I am a prisoner in my own body, an alive mind in a dead shell.

I cannot speak, eat or drink.

Swallowing is very difficult for me. I am fed by a feeding tube.

I have a hole in my neck, with a tracheotomy so I can breathe.

I am on a ventilator for 24 hours a day. I cannot cough up secretions, I need a special machine to vacuum out my lungs.

My jaw will lock up causing me to bite my tongue. I have to buzz for someone to pry my jaw open.

My life is lived in my mind, I lie in bed with just my thoughts and memories.

The highlight of my day is when I am sleeping at night. When I dream at night I am not paralyzed.

I have a special computer that enables me to type, speak, and go on the internet with just the movement of my eyes.

I am totally dependent on machines and other people, just to survive each day.

You would think that someone in this incomprehensible, debilitating, brutal situation would be seriously depressed, suicidal, crushed in spirit, aggressive and hateful. Incredibly, this was not the case. In fact, it was the exact opposite. David McClain was an outstanding example of a man whose spiritual growth and evolution were disproportionate to his imprisoned physical deterioration. In my experience, he is without a doubt the most spiritually evolved and faith sustained human being that I have had the privilege to know, either as a patient or in my own personal relationships.

The unassailable Christian faith of David McClain in his own articulate words:

As I travel this journey through the 'shadow of death', fear is NOT an option; my Savior and my King, Jesus Christ has carried me this far and will continue to carry me until that day that he calls me home to Glory. The weaker I become physically, the stronger I become spiritually. This 'raggedy old corruptible' body will someday be 'incorruptible'. This mortal body will put on immortality, then death will be swallowed by victory.

How great is that?!

In this world full of hatred, sadness and despair, there is a blessed hope through Jesus Christ that heaven is a 'reality'. Imagine a place where there will be no more tears, no more sorrow, no more crying, and no more pain. A place where earthly bodies will be transformed into glorified bodies, just like Jesus Christ when he rose from the grave.

It is a place where we will encounter loved ones and family and friends who have gone before and after us. We will live in Christ's radiant glory for ever and ever. Trust your heart and your life to him to be the love of your life.

David McClain soldiered on despite his debilitating physical handicap. His mind was constantly active and communicating thoughts in emails, blogs, on his Facebook page, and in computer-driven speech.

His courageous example of endurance is an inspiration to his friends and family. All that was made possible in large part by the care giving support and love showered on him by his wife, Donna, and his three devoted children.

Donna nursed him through his medical ordeal from the very beginning of his illness. She was with him at his first visit to my office and stood by him throughout his 12-year illness – whether it be handling emergencies with the failure of his respirator or emergency suctioning of his trachea or maintaining his hygiene or bathing him (with the help of a devoted aide), or even getting him ready for a special outside event at his daughter's graduation in a special van donated by caring friends.

His children Josh 29, Ben 27 and Kathleen 24 were a great strength, responsible for many of his needs. It is through them that he was last refreshed by their lives, and the outside world. The poignant relationship with his children is written in a poem entitled 'Daddy, read to me'.

Daddy please read to me. I love to hear your voice. Stories from the Bible are stories of my choice.

Daddy please sit next to me, let me hold your hand.

Daddy don't leave me. Please read to me again.

Then comes David's illness, which left him speechless and paralyzed, so the song poignantly shifts.

I lay in bed immobile, imprisoned in my sheets.

Terminally sick, I cannot speak, my days I cannot tell.

My arms and legs are paralyzed, alive throughout the day

When she walks by and she can hear me say

Kathleen please read to me, I love to hear your voice,

Stories from the Bible are stories of my choice.

Kathleen please sit next to me, let me hold your hand.

Kathleen read to me, please read to me again.

Life is but a vapor, soon I will go home

Then Kathleen I will read to you

Yes, you will hear my voice

I will sit next to you and I will hold your hand

I will never leave you

We are in the Promised Land

The song beautifully expresses the juxtaposition of a father's strength and his unconditional love, and his child's unshakeable trust. Then the dramatic change as the father is struck down and the child becomes the physical strength bonded with unconditional love. The father becomes the helpless child-like trusting dependent.

It is one of the mysteries of faith that at time of catastrophe it helps us sit with, suffer, endure and grow through such life situations. Faith that is rooted in profound grace, deeper than catastrophe that transcends survival and earthly sorrow and loss. It is through faith we hear the heartbeat of the world, of basic existence.

Mr David McClain and his children were remarkable in their continued devotion in the face of the enormous task of caring for David's survival.

In the difficult times when the task may have appeared to overwhelm them, it was David's pure, unbroken faith that sustained them all. This remarkable man survived 14 years – 10 years longer than the medical outcome predictions would approximate.

He evolved spiritually, and in many ways transcended his physical prison.

The 'dead shell' that he referred to as his mortal body, brought forth a faith so profound and inspiring that one can only stand in awe of the life force and the empowering spirituality that it generated. He survived so long because of the power of his faith and his humanity.

I have chosen to include the history of my patient David McClain because it illustrates the indomitable character of a man who will not give up on life. Like many patients in my practice, his tenacity, combined with his family's love and support, have seen him through his darkest hours. TBD infected patients often reflect similar strengths as did David (thought not to the extent of his profound disability), and are blessed with a steadfast faith that they will get well. Pharmaceuticals, herbals, nutraceuticals, homeopathic remedies, all have their place, but the unconditional love of a family and the unshakeable faith in a higher power triumph spiritually over the illness.

Chapter 27

Epilogue
The view from 80

Dr Bernard Raxlen

Virgil is credited with stating: *'Felix qui potuit rerum cognoscere causas,'* or, 'Fortunate is he who knows the causes of things'.

I used this quotation to open the introduction to Allie Cashel's first book, *Suffering the Silence: Chronic Lyme Disease in an Age of Denial*, an introduction she asked me to write at the end of 2014, over four years ago now. There was a sad, ironic coincidence to the timing of my writing. I finished my first draft on the night of November 17 2014, the very night of the death, at the age of 82, of Dr William Burgdorfer. As discoverer of the Borrelia spirochete that bears his name, Dr Burgdorfer will most certainly be included in the pantheon of those whose contributions have changed the course of medical history.

As I sat down to write the epilogue of this book, over four years after Dr Burgdorfer's death, I found myself wondering whether he would be satisfied with the progress that has been made in this field of TBD. Would he be disappointed that we still have difficulty in coming to a medical consensus on diagnosis or treatment?

Infected patients wonder why they aren't tested for Lyme, why their cases may have been missed, and which specialists they should seek out for treatment. Lost in the medical maze of Lyme disease, hundreds of thousands of individuals struggle every year to navigate their way back to health.

As has been stated by all of the authors contributing to this book, the denial of tick-borne illness is supported and maintained by an elaborate hierarchy of disinformation at multiple levels. In Gregory Bateson's language, the labyrinth is the journey through a dysfunctional medical system. As has been demonstrated here, laboratory testing is often inadequate or completely misleading. Patients who have negative blood test results aren't offered treatment. Positive results obtained by specialty labs are often ignored or even denigrated and often interpreted as 'false positive'. Worst of all, the IDSA guidelines do not recognize the existence of chronic Lyme disease, and therefore recommend only limited treatment.

This medical shortsightedness has been pervasive. Respected medical journals, from which physicians acquire up-to-date knowledge, are highly selective and tend to publish only research and opinion articles that support the CDC position. This rigid 'denial system' keeps medical wisdom truncated, doctors myopic and desperate patients, in many countries, untreated.

Each contributing author or advocate voice in this book has outlined a country-specific instance of this dysfunctional system we find ourselves in – the medical myopia of tick-borne disease.

When I look back on my history of almost 40 years with TBD, I see medical progress, even though unfair prejudices still exist. I do observe less medical myopia and more patients emerging positively from the debilitating maze of their disease experience. Many more patients are now armed with the correct diagnosis and are prescribed appropriate extended treatment protocols. There is, in addition, a massive presence on social media that dispenses helpful information (sometimes incorrectly). There are many local support groups that help patients feel connected to a common cause. There is an almost two-decades-old sophisticated medical caregiver organization, ILADS (International Lyme and Associated Diseases Society), dedicated to research and treatment of TBD. This organization supports like-minded doctors whose numbers grow yearly. ILADS embraces physicians from across all medical specialties, and hosts training programs for doctors as well as sponsoring yearly scientific conferences in both the US and Europe.

Non-profit citizen groups such as the Global Alliance (who merged with earlier citizen organizations such as Turn the Corner Foundation and Time for Lyme), LDA of New Jersey, and the Lyme Disease organization of Washington and California have raised millions of dollars for research to combat TBD. This active US citizen involvement, working toward the elimination of the scourge of tick-borne disease, has played a fundamental role in helping to develop new ways to combat TBD illnesses. In addition, this group of dedicated citizen organizations, many of whose members have themselves been afflicted, including their own family members, have organized town hall meetings and petitions and impacted local, state and federal government agencies to pass legislation in favor of those suffering from TBD. This in turn has persuaded a reluctant medical community to recognize, diagnose and treat TBD more carefully and substantially.

Max Planck, the famous German physicist and Nobel laureate, is reputed to have said that 'science advances one funeral at a time', meaning, of course, only when one generation of rigid adherents to a particular theory pass away, and only then, do new theories have a chance to take root and flourish. Hopefully in no more than another decade we will look back on the 'Lyme Wars' and marvel at how unnecessary it all was. What has been so hotly debated over a period of 40 years, roughly from 1980 to 2020, will appear self-evident and grounded scientifically in indisputable proof.

Hopefully, the next decade will be party to the combined efforts of dedicated patients and physicians cooperating in a concerted effort around the globe, to overcome not only the disease itself, but also the prejudice and short-sightedness of the 'locked system' that contributes to Medical Myopia and the bewildering labyrinth of TBD, in particular Lyme disease.

The view from 80

By the time this book is published, I will have passed my eightieth year on the planet. That includes 60 years (if you count medical school) studying and practicing medicine. Eight decades, 29,200 sunrises and sunsets (with a few eclipses thrown in). I find it remarkable how the years grew suddenly into a big pile of numbers, like single snowflakes accumulating into one huge snowdrift.

In spite of the snowdrift of years, I find it perfectly natural to subscribe to the illusion that I will go on living as if I was '20' again, with an 'ocean of time' ahead of me., and not a little frog pond. But I still experience the continuity of my self-system to be intact and consistent over all these years. I have had happy 'celebrations' at the 40, 50, 60 and 70 year markers. I shouldn't be, but I'm startled that my 80th year is upon me. I ask myself, would I do things differently in medicine? In particular, the chance encounter that led to my choosing to treat TBD?

As I have written, I slipped into the TBD field from psychiatry serendipitously, but once situated in this new 'sub-specialty', I have derived enormous satisfaction from my contact with and treatment of TBD patients. Hearing patients thank me for literally 'saving their lives' offers the greatest reward that I could receive. I also know that the physicians who have generously contributed to this book feel the same way.

Sigmund Freud MD on the occasion of his 80th birthday remarked in a letter to his colleague Ernst Jones MD:

> *what is the secret meaning of this celebrating the big round numbers of one's life? Surely a measure of triumph over the transistorizes of life, which, as we never forget, is ready to devour us. Then one rejoices with a sort of communal feeling that we are not made of such frail stuff as to prevent one of us victoriously resisting the hostile effects of life for 60, 70, or even 80 years. That is something one can understand and certainly agree with, but the celebration evidently makes sense only when the survivor can*

in spite of all wounds and scars join in as a hale fellow; it loses this sense when the individual is an invalid with whom there is no question of conviviality.

I consider myself fortunate to be one of those 'hale fellows' mentioned by Freud in this quotation. God willing, I will not be 'devoured by the transistorizes of life' quite yet. Hopefully I will be granted more time in which to practice medicine and in some small way help to eliminate the scourge of TBD that destroys patients' lives.

But as far as the corkscrew-shaped spiral bacteria *Borrelia burgdorferi* is concerned, the question is, will it evolve? Or, after so many millions of years, finally be eliminated as a life form? Or will it make the spectacular evolutionary journey along with mankind and change itself to become a more complex and advanced, vexing pathogen? My guess is that this immortal bacterium will survive long after we have perished as a species, finding novel hosts and vectors along the way to help it exist.

As Arno Karlen wrote in the final chapter of his book, *Biography of a Germ*:

Short of a doomsday nuclear event, the bacterium can outlive anything we can throw at it. I can picture only one of those cataclysms that at long intervals threaten much life on earth – the crash of asteroids, great heats and freezes, severe atmospheric and climate change, the rise and fall of seas. Heaven knows what these events will do to people. But in my mind's eye, I can see emerging from the rubble, a small wild mouse. On the mouse resides a tiny tick and, in the tick, there lazily turns a minute, slender spiral, hardy and elegant. Again, a survivor when so many of the planets' creatures have had their day and vanished.[184]

To my way of thinking, Borrelia has already achieved some of mankind's more elusive goals, such as 'immortality' through binary fission. Perhaps Borrelia has already achieved some sort of bacteriological 'bliss'. If we could tune into its vibrational energy, protected snug in some 'biofilm' quorum community. I wouldn't be the least bit surprised if its 'vibrational frequency' was actually a signal for 'Borrelia bliss'! As far as 'divine powers' are concerned, there is no contest. Borrelia has had a distinct and unfair advantage over Life as we know it on this planet. After all, it has had a half a billion years' actual head-start over us, eons before the concept of God existed in the minds of mankind, who had not yet been conceived.

Perhaps a few lines from Alfred Lord Tennyson's oft quoted great poem *Ulysses* would be in order as a closing thought, for me personally, and quite possibly for some of the other authors.

Old age had yet his honour and his toil;
Death closes all: but something ere the end,
Some work of noble note, may yet be done,
Not unbecoming men that strove with Gods. …
We are not now that strength which in old days
Moved earth and heaven, that which we are, we are;
One equal temper of heroic hearts,
Made weak by time and fate, but strong in will
To strive, to seek, to find, and not to yield.

References

Introduction

1. Pfeiffer MB (2018). *Lyme: The First Epidemic of Climate Change.* Washington DC: Island Press.

2. Asbrink E, Hovmark A. Successful cultivation of spirochetes from skin lesions of patients with erythema chronic migraines, Afzelius acrodermatis chronica atrophicans. *Acta Pathol Microbiol Immunol Sect B* 1985; 93: 161-163.

3. Stricker RB, Johnson L. Chronic Lyme Disease: Liberation from Lyme Denialism. *American Journal of Medicine* 2013; 126(8): e13 – e14.

4. CDC provides estimate of Americans diagnosed with Lyme disease each year. (2018, August 19). Retrieved from https://www.cdc.gov/media/releases/2013/p0819-lyme-disease.html

Chapter 1: Why is a psychiatrist treating Lyme disease?

5. Smith RC, Dwamena FC. Classification and Diagnosis of Patients with Medically Unexplained Symptoms. *Journal of General Internal Medicine* 2007; 22(5): 685-691. doi:10.1007/s11606-006-0067-2.

Chapter 2: The tick-borne disease commonalities

6. Bransfield R, Brand S, and Sheer V. Treatment of patients with persistent symptoms and a history of Lyme disease. *New England Journal of Medicine* 2001; 341: 1424-1425.

7. Cook MJ, Puri BK. Commercial test kits for detection of Lyme borreliosis: a meta-analysis of test accuracy. *Int J Gen Med* 2016; 2016(9): 427-440. doi 10.2147/ijgm.S122313.
8. Bakken LL, Callister SM, Wand PJ, Schell RF. Interlaboratory comparison of test results for detection of Lyme disease by 516 participants in the Wisconsin State Laboratory of Hygiene/College of American Pathologists Proficiency Testing Program. *Journal of Clinical Microbiology* 1997; 35(3): 537-543.
9. Pfeiffer MB (2018) *Lyme: The First Epidemic of Climate Change*. Washington, DC: Island Press.
10. Eddens T, Kaplan DJ, Anderson AJ, Nowalk AJ, Campfield BT. Insights from the Geographic Spread of the Lyme Disease Epidemic. *Clinical Infectious Diseases* 2019; 68(3): 426-434.
11. Hanincová K, Kurtenbach K, Diuk-Wasser M, Brei B, Fish D Epidemic spread of Lyme borreliosis, northeastern United States. *Emerging infectious Diseases* 2006; 12(4): 604.
12. Gulia-Nuss M, Nuss AB, Hill CA. Genomic insights into the Ixodes scapularis tick vector of Lyme disease. *Nature Communications* 2016; 7: 10507. DOI: 10.1038/ncomms10507
13. Smith Jr R, Lacombe EH, Morris SR, Holmes DW, Caporale DA. Role of bird migration in the long-distance dispersal of Ixodes dammini, the vector of Lyme disease. *Journal of Infectious Diseases* 1996; 174(1): 221-224.
14. Eddens T, Kaplan DJ, Anderson AJ, Nowalk AJ, Campfield BT. Insights from the Geographic Spread of the Lyme Disease Epidemic. *Clinical Infectious Diseases* 2019; 68(3): 426-434.
15. Ang CW, Notermans DW, Hommes M, Simoons-Smit AM, Herremans T. Large differences between test strategies for the detection of anti-Borrelia antibodies are revealed by comparing eight ELISAs and five immunoblots. *Eur J Clin Microbiol Infect Dis* 2011; 30(8): 1027-1032.
16. Weinstein ER, Rebman AW, Aucott JN, Johnson-Greene D, Bechtold KT. Sleep quality in well-defined Lyme disease: a clinical cohort study in Maryland. *Sleep* 2018; 41(5): zsy035.
17. Shadick NA, Phillips CB, Logigian EL et al. The long-term clinical outcomes of Lyme disease. A population-based retrospective cohort study. *Ann Intern Med* 1994 ; 121 : 905-908.
18. Oksi J, Marjamaki M, Nikoskelainen, Viljanen MK. Borrelia

burgdorferi detected by culture and PCR in clinical relapse of disseminated Lyme borreliosis. *Ann Med* 1999; 31: 225-232.

19. Hodzic E, Feng S, Holden K, Freet KJ, Barthold SW. Persistence of Borrelia burgdorferi following antibiotic treatment in mice. *Antimicrob Agents Chemother* 2008; 52: 1728-1736.

Chapter 3: Recognition of tick-borne disease

20. Dusenbery M, Rehmyer J. (2018, June 27). The Science Isn't Settled on Chronic Lyme. Retrieved from https://slate.com/technology/2018/06/the-science-isnt-settled-on-chronic-lyme.html
21. Clayton JL, Jones SG, Dunn JR, Schaffner W, Jones TF. Enhancing Lyme Disease Surveillance by Using Administrative Claims Data, Tennessee, USA. *Emerging Infectious Diseases* 2015; 21(9): 1632-1634. doi:10.3201/eid2109.150344.
22. Stricker RB, Johnson L. Chronic Lyme Disease: Liberation from Lyme Denialism. *American Journal of Medicine* 2013; 126(8): e13 – e14
23. Bransfield RC. A Physicians Opinion Survey of IDSA & ILADS Lyme Disease Guidelines [E-mail to the author]. (2014, August 12).
24. Dusenbery M, Rehmyer J. (2018, June 27). The Science Isn't Settled on Chronic Lyme. Retrieved from https://slate.com/technology/2018/06/the-science-isnt-settled-on-chronic-lyme.html

Chapter 4: Tick-borne disease – the basics

25. Adelson ME, Tilton RC, Cabets K, Eskow E, et al. Prevalence of Borrelia burgdorferi, Bartonella spp., Babesia microti and Anaplasma phagocytophilia in Ixodes. scapularis ticks collected in New Jersey. *J Clin Microbiol* 2004; 42(6): 2799-2801.

Chapter 5: The trouble with diagnosis

26. Alasel M, Keusgen M, Dassigner N. Development of a borreliosis assay: Mannan coated polyethylene sinter bodies as a new platform technology. *Analytical Biochemistry* 2017; 543. Retrieved from https://www.sciencedirect.com/science/article/pii/S0003269717304955
27. Theel ES. The Past, Present, and (Possible) Future of Serologic Testing for

Lyme Disease. *Journal of Clinical Microbiology* 2016; 54(5): 1191-1196.
28. Theel ES. The Past, Present, and (Possible) Future of Serologic Testing for Lyme Disease. *Journal of Clinical Microbiology* 2016; 54(5): 1191-1196.
29. Centers for Disease Control and Prevention. Lyme Disease: Diagnosis and Testing. Dec 21, 2018 www.cdc.gov/lyme/diagnosistesting/
30. Brorson O, Brorson SH. A rapid method for generating cystic forms of Borrelia burgdorferi, and their reversal to mobile spirochetes. *APMIS* 1998; 106: 1131-1141.

Chapter 7: Patient dismissal

31. Stricker RB. Counterpoint: long term antibiotic therapy improves persistent symptoms associated with Lyme disease. *Clin Infect Dis* 2007; 45: 149-157.
32. Liegner KB. Lyme disease: The Sensible Pursuit of Answers. *J Clin Microbiol* 1993; 31: 1961-1963.
33. Statement for the House Foreign Affairs Committee Africa, Global Health and Human Rights Subcommittee's Hearing on Global Challenges in Diagnosing and Managing Lyme Disease — Closing Knowledge Gaps[PDF]. (2012, July 17). Submitted by the Infectious Diseases Society of America.
34. Lyme Disease and other Tick-Borne Diseases[PDF]. (2017, February 23). Aetna.

Chapter 8: Treatment – the nuts and bolts

35. DeLong AK, Blossom B, Maloney EL, Phillips SE. Antibiotic retreatment of Lyme disease in patients with persistent symptoms: a biostatistical review of randomized, placebo-controlled, clinical trials. *Contemp Clin Trials* 2012; 33: 1132-1142.
36. Lewis K. Persister cells, dormancy and infectious disease. *Nature* 2007; 5. doi: 10.1038/nrmicro1557
37. Meriläinen L, Herranen A, Schwarzbach A, Gilbert L. Morphological and biochemical features of Borrelia burgdorferi pleomorphic forms. *Microbiology* 2015; 161. 516-527.
38. Krupp LB, Masr D, Schqartz J, Coyle PK, Langenback IJ, Fernquist SK. Cognitive functioning in late Lyme borreliosis. *Arch Neurol* 1999; 48: 1125-1129.

39. Brorson O, Brorson SH. Transformation of cystic forms of Borrelia burgdorferi to normal, mobile spirochetes. *Infection* 1997; 25: 240-246.
40. Murgia CM. Induction of cystic forms by different stress conditions in Borrelia burgdorferi. *APMIS* 2004; 112: 57-62.
41. Brorson O, Brorson SH. In vitro conversion of Borrelia burgdorferi to cystic forms in spinal fluid, and transformation to mobile spirochetes by incubation in BSK-H medium. *Infection* 1998; 26: 144–150. doi:10.1007/BF02 771839
42. Brorson O, Brorson SH. Transformation of cystic forms of Borrelia burgdorferi to normal, mobile spirochetes, *Infection* 1997; 25: 240-246.
43. Horowitz R (2013) *Why Can't I Get Better? Solving the Mystery of Lyme and Chronic Disease*. St Martin's Press.
44. Cusick MF, Libbey JE, Fujinami RS. Molecular Mimicry as a Mechanism of Autoimmune Disease. *Clinical Reviews in Allergy & Immunology* 2012; 42(1): 102-111. doi:10.1007/s12016-011-8294-7.
45. Lyme Disease and other Tick-Borne Diseases [PDF]. (2017, February 23). Aetna.
46. Horowitz R. (2013). *Why Can't I Get Better? Solving the Mystery of Lyme and Chronic Disease*. St Martin's Press.
47. The Clinical Assessment, Treatment, and Prevention of Lyme Disease, Human Granulocytic Anaplasmosis, and Babesiosis. (2006). Retrieved from www.idsociety.org/Topics_of_Interest/Lyme_Disease/Public_Policy/Lyme_Disease/
48. Keller A, Graefen A, Ball M, et al. New insights into the Tyrolean Iceman's origin and phenotype as inferred by whole-genome sequencing. *Nature Communications* 2012; 3: 698. doi:10.1038/ncomms1701.
49. Horowitz R (2013) *Why Can't I Get Better? Solving the Mystery of Lyme and Chronic Disease*. St Martin's Press.
50. Burrascano J. Advanced topics in Lyme disease: diagnostic hints and treatment guidelines for Lyme and other tick-borne illnesses. [PDF]. International Lyme and Associated Diseases Society, October 2008. www.researchednutritionals.com/dr-burrascanos-advanced-topics-in-lyme-disease/
51. ILADS Conference 2018. www.ilads.org/ilads-conference/chicago-2018/
52. Stricker RB. Counterpoint: long term antibiotic therapy improves persistent symptoms associated with Lyme disease. *Clin Infect Dis* 2007; 45: 149-157.

53. Horowitz R (2013) *Why Can't I Get Better? Solving the Mystery of Lyme and Chronic Disease.* St Martin's Press.
54. Zhou G, Shi Q, Huang X-M, Xie XB. The three bacterial lines of defense against antimicrobial agents. *International Journal of Molecular Sciences* 2015; 16: 21711-21733.

Chapter 9: Identity, self-esteem and Lyme patienthood

55. Wang G, Liveris D, Brei B, et al. Real-time PCR for simultaneous detection and quantification of Borrelia burgdorferi in field-collected Ixodes scapularis ticks from the Northeastern United States. *Appl Environ Microbiol* 2003; 69(8):4561-4565.
56. Macrae CN, Moran JM, Heatherton TF, Banfield JF, Kelley WM. Medial prefrontal activity predicts memory for self. *Cerebral Cortex* 2004; 14(6): 647-654 .
57. Damasio A, Carvalho GB. The nature of feelings: evolutionary and neurobiological origins. *Nature Reviews Neuroscience* 2013; 14(2): 143.
58. Klemm WR. Neural representations of the sense of self. *Advances in Cognitive Psychology* 2011; 7: 16-30.

Chapter 10: The family system response to tick-borne disease

59. Leonard BE. The concept of depression as a dysfunction of the immune system. *Current Immunology Reviews* 2010; 6(3): 205-212.
59. Buchwald A. Ein Fall von diffuser idiopathischer Hautatrophie. *Arch Dermatol Syph* 1983; 10: 553-556. http://link.springer.com/article/10.1007%2FBF01833474?LI=true#page-1. 60. Lyme Disease and other Tick-Borne Diseases [PDF]. (2017, February 23). Aetna.
61. Sigal L. The Lyme disease controversy: social and financial costs of misdiagnosis and mismanagement. *Arch Int Med* 1996; 156: 1493–1500.

Chapter 13: *The Biography of a Germ*

62. Karlen A (2001) *Biography of a Germ.* New York: Anchor Books.

Chapter 14: From New York to the UK

63. Buchwald A. Ein Fall von diffuser indiopathischer Hautatrophie. *Arch Dermatol Syph* 1883; 10: 553-556 (http://link.springer.com/article/10.1007%2FBF01833474?L=true#page-1
64. Keller A, Graefen A, Ball M, Matzas M et al. New insights into Tyrolean Iceman's origin and phenotype as inferred by whole-genome sequencing. *Nat Comms* 2012; 3: 698. DOI: 10.1038/ncomms1701.
65. Matuschka FR, Ohlenbusch A, Eiffert H, Richter D, Spielman A. Characteristics of Lyme disease spirochetes in archived European ticks. *J Infect Dis* 1996; 174: 424–426.
66. Obasi O. Erythema chronicum migrans. *Br J Dermatol* 1977; 97(4): 459. doi:10.1111/j.1365-2133.1977.tb14260.x.
67. Hubbard MJ, Baker AS, Cann KJ. Distribution of Borrelia burgdorferi s.l. spirochaete DNA in British ticks (Argasidae and Ixodidae) since the 19th century, assessed by PCR. *Med Vet Entomol* 1998; 12: 89–97. doi:10.1046/j.1365-2915.1998.00088.x
68. Williams D, Rolles C, White J. Lyme disease in a Hampshire child-medical curiosity or beginning of an epidemic? BMJ(Clin Res Ed) 1986; 292: 1560.
69. Kurtenbach K, De Michelis S, Sewell H-S, et al. Distinct combinations of Borrelia burgdorferi sensu lato genospecies found in individual questing ticks from Europe. *Appl Environ Microbiol* 2001; 67(10): 4926-4929. http://opus.bath.ac.uk/4334/.
70. Hansford KM, Fonville M, Jahfari S, Sprong H, Medlock JM. Borrelia miyamotoi in host-seeking Ixodes ricinus ticks in England. *Epidemiol Infect* 2015; 143(5): 1079-1087. www.ncbi.nlm.nih.gov/pubmed/25017971.
71. Sato K, Takano A, Konnai S, et al. Human Infections with Borrelia miyamotoi, Japan. *Emerg Infect Dis* 2014; 20(8): 1391-1394. doi:10.3201/eid2008.131761.
72. Centers for Disease Control and Prevention. CDC provides estimate of Americans diagnosed with Lyme disease each year. CDC Media Relations Press Release Monday, August 19, 2013. www.cdc.gov/media/releases/2013/p0819-lyme-disease.html.
73. Lindgren E, Jaenson TGT. Lyme borreliosis in Europe : influences of climate and climate change, epidemiology, ecology and adaptation measures. In: Menne B, Ebi KL (eds) *World Health*

2006; EU/04/5046. www.euro.who.int/__data/assets/pdf_file/0006/96819/E89522.pdf.

74. Müller I, Mh F, Poggensee G, Scharnetzky E, Kp H. Evaluating Frequency , Diagnostic Quality and Cost of Lyme Borreliosis Testing in Germany : A Retrospective Model Analysis.*Clin Dev Immunol* 2012; 2012:595427. . doi: 10.1155/2012/595427

75. Topping A. GP consultations too short for complex cases, says doctors' leader. *The Guardian*. www.theguardian.com/society/2017/feb/07/gps-consultation-times-too-short-for-complex-cases-says-doctors-leader. Published 2017. (Accessed 10 April 2019.)

76. Dixon J, Lewis R, Rosen R, Finlayson B, Gray D (2004) *Managing Chronic Disease: What Can We Learn from the US Experience?* The King's Fund: London, UK. www.kingsfund.org.uk%5Cnwww.kingsfund.org.uk/publications.

77. Leeflang M, Ang C, Berkhout J, et al. The diagnostic accuracy of serological tests for Lyme borreliosis : a systematic review and meta-analysis . *BMC Infect Dis* 2016; 16(140): 1-17. doi:10.1186/s12879-016-1468-4.

78. Zeller H, Van Bortel W for ECDC. *A Systematic Literature Review on the Diagnosis Accuracy of Serological Tests for Lyme Borreliosis*. Stockholm: European Centre for Disease Prevention and Control; 2016. https://ecdc.europa.eu/sites/portal/files/media/en/publications/Publications/lyme-borreliosis-diagnostic-accuracy-serological-tests-systematic-review.pdf

79. Cook MJ, Puri BK. Commercial test kits for the detection of Lyme borreliosis: a meta-analysis of test accuracy. *Int J Gen Med* 2016; 9: 427-440. doi: https://doi.org/10.2147/IJGM.S122313.

80. Cook MJ, Puri BK. Application of Bayesian decision-making to laboratory testing for Lyme disease and comparison with testing for HIV. *Int J Gen Med* 2017; 10: 113-123. www.dovepress.com/articles.php?article_id=32303.

81. Cook M, Puri B. Update to: Application of Bayesian decision-making to laboratory testing for Lyme disease and comparison with testing for HIV. *Int J Gen Med* 2017; 10: 291-292. doi: 10.2147/IJGM.S145134.

82. Assoc of State and Territorial Public Health Laboratory Directors. Proceedings of the 2nd National Conference on Serologic Diagnosis of Lyme Disease. In: *Second National Conference on Serologic Diagnosis of Lyme Disease*. Dearborn, Michigan; 1994: 1-111.

83. Kahn DW, Malawista SE. Lyme disease: Recommendations for diagnosis and treatment. *Ann Intern Med* 1991; 114:472. DOI:10.7326/0003-4819-114-6-472.

84. Wormser GP, Nadelman RB, Dattwyler RJ, et al. Practice Guidelines for the Treatment of Lyme Disease. *Clin Infect Dis* 2000; 3(1): S1-14. doi: 10.1086/512462.

85. The ILADS Working Group. Lyme and Associated Diseases Society Evidence-based Guidelines for the Management of Lyme Disease. *Expert Rev Anti Infect Ther* 2004; 2(1).

86. Feder HM, Johnson BJB, O'Connell S, Shapiro ED, Steere AC, Wormser GP. A Critical Appraisal of Chronic Lyme Disease. *N Engl J Med* 2007; 357(14): 1422-1430. doi:10.1056/NEJMra072023.

87. Wormser GP, Dattwyler RJ, Shapiro ED, et al. The clinical assessment, treatment, and prevention of Lyme disease, human granulocytic anaplasmosis, and babesiosis: clinical practice guidelines by the Infectious Diseases Society of America. *Clin Infect Dis* 2006; 43(9): 1089-1134. doi:10.1086/508667.

88. Prautzch H, Borreliose-gesellschaft D. DBG Objections to the IDSA Lyme Guidelines. Karlsruhe, Germany: 2009. www.lymenet.de/literatur/dbg_idsa_statement.pdf.

89. Lyme Disease Action (2011) Comment on the British Infection Association's Position Statement on Lyme Borreliosis. www.lymediseaseaction.org.uk/wp-content/uploads/2011/08/LDA-on-BIA.pdf.

90. Shaneyfelt T. In Guidelines We Cannot Trust. *Arch Intern Med* 2012; 172(21): 1633-1634. doi:10.1001/2013.

91. Lee DH, Vielemeyer O. Analysis of overall level of evidence behind Infectious Diseases Society of America practice guidelines. *Arch Intern Med* 2011; 171(1): 18-22. doi:10.1001/archinternmed.2010.482.

92. Wormser GP, Baker PJ, O'Connell S, Pachner AR, Schwartz I, Shapiro ED. Critical Analysis of Treatment Trials of Rhesus Macaques Infected with Borrelia burgdorferi Reveals Important Flaws in Experimental Design. *Vector Borne Zoonotic Disease* 2012; 12. doi:10.1089/vbz.2012.1012

93. Ford S. Draft guidance drawn up to "spot and treat" Lyme disease. *Nursing Times* 2017; 26 September. www.nursingtimes.net/news/primary-care/draft-guidance-drawn-up-to-spot-and-treat-lyme-disease/7021404.article.

94. Sims I. GPs advised not to rule out Lyme disease despite lack of tick bite. *Pulse* 2017, 25 September. www.pulsetoday.co.uk/news/clinical-news/gps-advised-not-to-rule-out-lyme-disease-despite-lack-of-tick-bite/20035346.article#.WdDntq2dobI.facebook.

95. Faust S. Membership of Lyme Disease Guideline Committee. 2018, 11 April. www.nice.org.uk/guidance/ng95/evidence/membership-of-the-guideline-committee-pdf-4792274895 (accessed 12 April 2019)

96. NICE. Lyme disease Guideline 2018, April and October. www.nice.org.uk/guidance/ng95 (accessed 12 April 2019)

97. Cruickshank M, O'Flynn N, Faust SN. Lyme disease: Summary of NICE guidance. *BMJ* 2018; 361: 1–6. doi:10.1136/bmj.k1261

98. World Health Organization. *The Treatment of Tuberculosis Guidelines* 4th edition. Geneva, Switzerland: World Health Organization; 2010. www.who.int/tb/publications/2010/9789241547833/en/

99. World Health Organization. *Guidelines for the Diagnosis, Treatment, and Prevention of Leprosy. Executive summary*. Geneva, Switzerland: WHO; 2018. www.who.int/neglected_diseases/news/WHO-to-publish-first-guidelines-on-leprosy-diagnosis/en/

100. Brunton G, Sutcliffe K, Hinds K et al (2017) Stakeholder experiences of the diagnosis of Lyme disease A systematic review. London: EPPI-Centre, Social Sciences Research Unit, UCL Institute of Education, University College London. https://eppi.ioe.ac.uk/cms/Portals/0/PDF reviews and summaries/Lyme disease stakeholder experiences 2017 Brunton.pdf?ver=2018-04-23-155309-640

101. Bloor K. Lyme and Tick-borne Infections Patient Survey. 2014. http://lymeresearchuk.org/wp-content/uploads/2012/04/prof-diag-final-WPress.pdf

102. Auwaerter PG, Bakken JS, Dattwyler RJ, et al. Antiscience and ethical concerns associated with advocacy of Lyme disease. *Lancet Infect Dis* 2011; 11(9): 713-719. doi:10.1016/S1473-3099(11)70034-2.

103. Schmutzhard E, Pallua A, Stanek G, Pletschette M, Hirschl AM, Schlögl R, et al. Infections following tickbites. Tick-borne encephalitis and lyme borreliosis — A prospective epidemiological study from tyrol. *Infection* 1988; 16: 269–272. doi:10.1007/BF01645068

104. Morgan-Capner P, Cutler S., Wright DJ., Hamlet N, Nathwani D, Ho-Yen D., et al. Borrelia burgdorferi infection in UK workers at risk

of tick bites. *Lancet*; 1989; 8: 789. doi:10.1016/S0140-6736(89)92812-3

105. Arzouni J, Laveran M, Beytout J, Ramousse O, Raolt D. Comparison of Western Blot and microimmunofluorescence as tools for Lyme disease seroepidemiology. *Eur J Epidemiol* 1993; 9: 269–273.
106. Ghionni A, Nuti M, Lillini E, Crovatto M, Santini GF, Polato D, et al. Infections in an Alpine environment: Antibodies to Hantaviruses, Leptospira, Rickettsiae, and Borrelia burgdorferi in defined Italian populations. *Am J Trop Med Hyg* 1993; 48: 20–25. doi:10.4269/ajtmh.1993.48.20
107. Kuiper H, de Jongh BM, Nauta AP, Houweling H, Wiessing LG, van Charante AW, et al. Lyme borreliosis in Dutch forestry workers. *J Infect* 1991; 23: 279–286. www.ncbi.nlm.nih.gov/pubmed/1753136
108. Fahrer H, Sauvain MJ, Zhioua E, Van Hoecke C, Gern LE. Longterm survey (7 years) in a population at risk for Lyme borreliosis: What happens to the seropositive individuals? *Eur J Epidemiol* 1998; 14: 117–123. doi:10.1023/A:1007404620701
109. Steere AC, Malawista SE, Snydman DR, Shope RE, Andiman WA, Ross MR, et al. Lyme Arthritis: An epidemic of oligoarticular arthritis in children and adults in three Connecticut communities. *Arthritis Rheum* 1977; 20: 7–17. doi:10.1002/art.1780200102

Chapter 15: Lyme disease in Ireland

110. Johnson L, Stricker RB. The Infectious Diseases Society of America Lyme guidelines: a cautionary tale about the development of clinical practice guidelines. *Philosophy, Ethics, and Humanities in Medicine : PEHM* 2010; 5: 9. doi:10.1186/1747-5341-5-9.
111. www.hpsc.ie/a-z/vectorborne/lymedisease/informationforthepublic/ (accessed 10 April 2019)
112. Estrada-Peña A, Cutler S, Potkonjak A, Vassier-Tussaut M, Van Bortel W, Zeller H, Fernández-Ruiz N, Mihalca AD An updated meta-analysis of the distribution and prevalence of Borrelia burgdorferi s.l. in ticks in Europe. *Int J Health Geogr* 2018; 17(1): 41. doi: 10.1186/s12942-018-0163-7.
113. Ostfeld RS, Brunner JL. Climate change and Ixodes tick-borne diseases of humans. *Philos Trans R Soc Lond B Biol Sci* 2015; 370(1665). pii: 20140051. doi: 10.1098/rstb.2014.0051. Review. http://ticktalkireland.org/testing.html

114. www.eaneurology.org/fileadmin/user_upload/guidline_papers/EFNS_guideline_2010_European_lyme_neuroborreliosis.pdf
115. Mygland Å, Ljøstad U, Fingerle Y, Rupprecht T, et al. EFNS guidelines on the diagnosis and management of European Lyme neuroborreliosis. *European Journal of Neurology* 2010; 17:8-16.

Chapter 16: From Lyme disease to crypto-infections: the story of Lyme in France

116. ESGBOR (www.escmid.org/research_projects/study_groups/lyme_borreliosis/) (accessed 11 April 2019)
117. Institute of Medicine, National Guideline Clearinghouse https://lymediseaseassociation.org/news/national-guideline-clearinghouse-website-to-shut-down-in-july/
118. Haut Conseil de la Santé Publique. Mieux connaître la borréliose de Lyme pour mieux la prévenir. 29 January 2010 : www.hcsp.fr/Explore.cgi/avisrapports- domaine?clefr=138
119. Haut Conseil de la Santé Publique. Borréliose de Lyme. Etat des connaissances. 28 March 2014 : www.hcsp.fr/Explore.cgi/avisrapportsdomaine?clefr=465
120. Nicolle C. *Destin des Maladies Infectieuses*. Paris, Librairie Félix Alcan, 1933; reprinted by the Association des Anciens élèves de l'Institut Pasteur, Paris, France Lafayette edition, 1993.
121. Perronne C. (2018) *La Vérité sur la Maladie de Lyme* (The Truth about Lyme Disease). Paris, Odile Jacob.
122. Haut Conseil de la Santé Publique. Borréliose de Lyme. Etat des connaissances. 28 March 2014 : www.hcsp.fr/Explore.cgi/avisrapportsdomaine?clefr=465 (accessed 10 April 2019)
123. Vayssier-Taussat M, Moutailler S, Féménia F, Raymond P, et al. Identification of novel zoonotic activity of Bartonella spp. *Emerg Infect Dis* 2016, 22(3): 457-462.
124. Perronne C. Lyme and associated tick-borne diseases : Global challenges in the context of a public health threat. *Front Cell Infect Microbiol* 2014; 4: 74.
125. Cook MJ, Puri BK. Commercial test kits for detection of Lyme borreliosis: a meta-analysis of test accuracy. *Int J Gen Med* 2016; 18(9); 427-440.
126. http://ecdc.europa.eu/en/publications/Publications/lyme-

borreliosis-diagnostic-accuracy-serological-tests-systematic-review.pdf

127. Haut Conseil de la Santé Publique. Borréliose de Lyme. Etat des connaissances. 28 March 2014 : www.hcsp.fr/Explore.cgi/avisrapportsdomaine?clefr=465
128. French Federation Against Tick-borne Diseases http://ffmvt.org (accessed 11 April 2019)
129. The documentary When ticks attack! aired on Tuesday, May 20, 2014 on the channel France 5 at 20:35 Prime Time.
130. Lenglet R, Perrin C. *L'affaire de la maladie de Lyme. Une enquête*. Arles, Actes Sud, 2016.
131. Lyme: the invisible epidemic French tv special. Aired on Canal Plus October 2014.
132. Albertat J (2012) *Maladie de Lyme. Mon parcours pour retrouver la santé* Thierry Souccar Publisher, Vergèze, France.
133. Cook MJ, Puri BK. Commercial test kits for detection of Lyme borreliosis: a meta-analysis of test accuracy. *Int J Gen Med* 2016; 18(9): 427-440.
134. www.has-sante.fr/portail/upload/docs/application/pdf/2018-06/reco266_rbp_borreliose_de_lyme_cd_2018_06_13__recommandations.pdf (accessed 11 April 2019)
135. www.has-sante.fr/portail/upload/docs/application/pdf/2018-06/reco266_rbp_borreliose_de_lyme_cd_2018_06_13__recommandations.pdf (accessed 11 April 2019)
136. https://ecdc.europa.eu/en/publications-data/ecdc-tool-prioritisation-infectious-disease-threats
137. www.hhs.gov/sites/default/files/tbdwg-report-to-congress-2018.pdf?fbclid=IwAR1u5BTMGMUMCIdMOfudGAqChW1psJL42117 6FXWWn4u-YYh2edmRR0LHyw (accessed 11 April 2019)
138. Perronne C (2017) *La Vérité sur la Maladie de Lyme* (The Truth about Lyme Disease) Paris, Odile Jacob
139. Guyatt GH, Oxman AD, Vist GE et al. GRADE: an emerging consensus on rating quality of evidence and strength of recommendations. *BMJ* 2008; 336 : 924-926.

Chapter 17: Lyme and tick-borne disease in Spain

140. www.eea.europa.eu/data-and-maps/indicators/vector-borne-diseases-1/assessment

141. Alonso FM. Lyme Disease, is it so uncommon? *Semergen* 2012; 38: 118-121.

142. www.researchgate.net/figure/272076390_fig4_Figure-1-Distribution-of-Ixodes-ricinus-and-Rhipicephalus-sanguineus-in-Europe-The (European Center for Disease Control, Jan 2015)

143. www.researchgate.net/figure/272076390_fig4_Figure-1-Distribution-of-Ixodes-ricinus-and-Rhipicephalus-sanguineus-in-Europe-The (European Center for Disease Control, Jan 2015)

144. Ros-García et al. Monitoring piroplasms infection in three cattle farms in Minorca (Balearic Islands, Spain) with previous history of clinical piroplasmosis. *Vet Parasitol* 2012; 190: 3-4.

145. Fernandez de Mera et al. Spotted Fever Group Rickettsiae in Questing Ticks, Central Spain. *Emerg Infect Dis* 2013; 19(7): 1163-1165.

146. Camacho AT et al. Theileria (Babesia) equi and Babesia caballi Infections in Horses in Galicia, Spain. *Trop Anim Health Prod* 2005; 37(4): 293-302.

Chapter 18: Diagnosis and treatment of tick-borne disease in Germany

147. Epidemiologisches Bulletin Nr. 17/2017, Robert Koch Institut. www.rki.de/DE/Content/Infekt/EpidBull/Archiv/2018/Ausgaben/17-18.pdf?

148. Sapi E, Kaur N, Anyanwu S, et al. Evaluation of in-vitro antibiotic susceptibility of different morphological forms of Borrelia burgdorferi. *Infect Drug Resist* 2011; 4: 97-113.

149. Gabriele Multhoff (2009) Activation of natural killer cells by heat shock protein 70. *International Journal of Hyperthermia* 2009; 25(3): 169-175. DOI:10.1080/02656730902902001

150. Newman EA, Eisen L, Eisen RJ, Fedorova N, Hasty JM, et al. Borrelia burgdorferi Sensu Lato Spirochetes in Wild Birds in Northwestern California: Associations with Ecological Factors, Bird Behavior and Tick Infestation. *PLOS ONE* 2015; 10(2): e0118146. https://doi.org/10.1371/journal.pone.0118146

Chapter 19: A summary of the European situation and new testing Tickplex and ELISpot

151. Lehman PV et al.: Unique Strengths of ELISpot for T Cell Diagnostics. In: Kalyuzhny AE. Handbook of ELISpot: Methods and Protocols, Methods in Molecular Biology, Vol. 792. 2nd Ed: Springer; 2012: 3-23

Chapter 20: Tick-borne diseases in Australia – different things to different people

152. www.abs.gov.au/AUSSTATS/abs@.nsf/Lookup/4102.0Main+Features20Sep+2010
153. Barker SC, Walker AR. Ticks of Australia. The species that infest domestic animals and humans. *Zootaxa* 2014: 3816:1-144. doi: 10.11646/zootaxa.3816.1.1
154. Fotso Fotso A, Drancourt M. Laboratory Diagnosis of Tick-Borne African Relapsing Fevers: Latest Developments. *Front Public Health* 2015; 3: 254. doi: 10.3389/fpubh.2015.00254. eCollection 2015.
155. Dickinson GS, Allugupalli KR. Deciphering the role of toll-like receptors in humoral responses to Borreliae. *Front Biosci* 2012; 4: 699-712.
156. Loh SM, Gillett A, Ryan U, Irwin P, Oskam C. Molecular characterization of 'Candidatus Borrelia tachyglossi' (family Spirochaetaceae) in echidna ticks, Bothriocroton concolor. *Int J Syst Evol Microbiol* 2017; 67(4): 1075-1080. doi: 10.1099/ijsem.0.001929
157. Mackerras MJ. *The Haematozoa of Australian Mammals.* 1959 105-261
158. Carley JG, Pope JH. A new species of Borrelia (B. queenslandica) from Rattus villosissimus in Queensland. *Aust J Exp Biol Med Sci* 1962; 40: 255-261.
159. Stewart A, Glass J, Patel A, Watt G, Gripps A, Clancy R. Lyme arthritis in the Hunter valley. *Med. J Aust* 1982; 1: 139.
160. McCrossin I. Lyme disease on the NSW south coast. *Med J Aust* 1986; 144(13): 724-725.
161. Lawrence RH, Bradbury R, Cullen JS. Lyme disease on the NSW central coast. *Med J Aust* 1986; 145(7): 364.
162. Piesman J, Stone BF. Vector competence of the Australian paralysis tick, Ixodes holocyclus, for the Lyme disease spirochete Borrelia burgdorferi. *Int J Parasitol* 1991; 21(1): 109-111.

163. Russell RC, Doggett SL, Munro R, Ellis J, Avery D, Hunt C, Dickeson D. Lyme disease: a search for a causative agent in ticks in south-eastern Australia. *Epidemiol Infect* 1994; 112(2): 375-384.
164. Wills MC, Barry RD. Detecting the cause of Lyme disease in Australia. *Med J Aust* 1991; 155(4): 275.
165. Hudson BJ, Stewart M, Lennox VA, Fukunaga M, Yabuki M, Macorison H, Kitchener-Smith J. Culture-positive Lyme borreliosis. *Med J Aust* 1998; 168(10): 500-502.
166. www.health.gov.au/internet/main/publishing.nsf/Content/ohp-cacld-lyme-disease.htm#terms.
167. http://health.gov.au/lyme-disease#scoping
168. www.aph.gov.au/Parliamentary_Business/Committees/Senate/Community_Affairs/Lymelikeillness45/Final_Report)
169. McManus M, Cincotta A. Effect of Borrelia on the host immune system: Possible consequences for diagnostics. 2015 *Adv Integ Medicine* 2015; 2(2): 81-89.
170. Gofton AW, Margos G, Fingerle V, Hepner S, Loh SM, Ryan U, Irwin P, Oskam CL. Genome-wide analysis of Borrelia turcica and 'Candidatus Borrelia tachyglossi' shows relapsing fever-like genomes with unique genomic links to Lyme disease Borrelia. *Infect Genet Evol* 2018; 66: 72-81. doi: 10.1016/j.meegid.2018.09.013. Epub 2018 Sep 18.
171. https://nhmrc.gov.au/about-us/news-centre/3-million-tick-bite-medical-research
172. http://karlmcmanusfoundation.org.au/human-rights-violations-of-people-suffering-tick-borne-illness/

Chapter 22: Lyme in Mexico

173. Parry, W. (2012, February 28). Iceman Mummy May Hold Earliest Evidence of Lyme Disease. www.livescience.com/18704-oldest-case-lyme-disease-spotted-iceman-mummy.html (accessed 12 April 2019)
174. www.lymedisease.org/lyme-basics/co-infections/about-co-infections/ (accessed 12 April 2019)
175. Gordillo Pérez G, Solórzano Santos F. Lyme's disease. Experience in Mexican children. *Medical Bulletin of the Children's Hospital of Mexico* 2010; 67(2): 164-176. (Retrieved on April 8, 2019, from http://www.scielo.org.mx/scielo.php?script=sci_

arttext&pid=S1665-11462010000200010&lng=es&tlng=es. First cases confirmed in Medico 1991)

176. Meléndez MG, Taylor CS, Alanís JC. Enfermedad de Lyme: Actualizaciones. *Gaceta Médica de México* 2014; 150: 84-95. doi: www.anmm.org.mx/GMM/2014/n1/GMM_150_2014_1_084-095.pdf

177. Taylor CMS, Gonzalez MSF, Pedraza IJC, Palacios CKS, Elizondo MAG. Enfermedad de Lyme. *Medicinea Universitaria* 2007; 9(34): 24-32. www.medigraphic.com/pdfs/meduni/mu-2007/mu071f.pdf (accessed 12 April 2019)

178. Gordillo-Pérez G, Torres J, Solórzano-Santos F, Garduño-Bautista V, Tapia-Conyer R, Muñoz O. Seroepidemiological study of Lyme borreliosis in Mexico City and the northeast of the Mexican Republic. *Public Health of Mexico* 2003; 45 (5): 351-355. (Retrieved on April 8 2019 from www.scielo.org.mx/scielo.php?script=sci_arttext&pid=S0036-36342003000500004&lng=es&tlng=es.)

179. Gordillo-Pérez G, Torres J, Solórzano-Santos F, de Martino S, Lipsker D, Velázquez E, Jaulhac B. Borrelia burgdorferi infection and cutaneous Lyme disease, Mexico. *Emerging Infectious Diseases* 2007; 13(10): 1556–1558. doi:10.3201/eid1310.060630

180. Gordillo-Pérez G, Torres J, Solórzano-Santos F, Cedillo R, Tapia Conyer R, Muñoz O. Serologic Evidences Suggesting the Presence of Borrelia burgdorferi Infection in Mexico. *Archives of Medical Research* 1999; 30: 64-68. DOI: 10.1016/S0188-0128(98)00015-3.

181. Gordillo-Pérez G, Solórzano-Santos F. Enfermedad de Lyme. Experiencia en ninos mexicanos. (Lyme disease. Experience in Mexican children) *Tema Pedriatrico: Bol Med Hosp Infant Mex* 2010; 67: 164-176. (Retrieved from www.medigraphic.com/pdfs/bmhim/hi-2010/hi102j.pdf)

182. www.cenetec.salud.gob.mx/descargas/gpc/CatologoMaestro/588_GPC_ExtantemasInfecciososenlainfancia/588GRR.pdf]

Chapter 25: Lyme as teacher and guide

183. Sontag S (2001) *Illness as Metaphor* USA: Picador.

Chapter 27: Epilogue: the view from 80

184. Karlen A (2001) *Biography of a Germ* New York: Anchor Books.

Appendices

Bibliography

Asch ES, Bujak DI, Weiss M et al. Lyme disease: an infectious and postinfectious syndrome. *J Rheumatol* 1994; 21: 454-461.

Azria E. The Human Element vs. the Standardization of Medical Care. Books and Ideas , 5 June 2014. www.booksandideas.net/The-Human-Element-vs-the.html (accessed 9 April 2019)

Barthold SW, Hodzic E, Imai DM et al. Ineffectiveness of tigecycline against persistent Borrelia burgdorferi. *Antimicrob Agents Chemother* 2010; 54: 643-651.

Brorson O, Brorson SH. In vitro conversion of Borrelia burgdorferi to cystic forms in spinal fluid, and transformation to mobile spirochetes by incubation in BSK-H medium. *Infection* 1998; 26: 144–150. doi:10.1007/BF02 771839

Brorson O, Brorson SH. Transformation of cystic forms of *Borrelia burgdorferi* to normal, mobile spirochetes, *Infection* 1997; 25: 240-6

Berende A, ter Hofstede HJM, Vos FJ, van Midendorp H., Vogelaar ML, Tromp M et al. Cost-effectiveness of longer-term versus shorter-term provision of antibiotics in patients with persistent symptoms attributed to Lyme disease. *N Engl J Med* 2016 ; 374: 1209-1220.

Cairns V, Godwin J. Post-Lyme borreliosis syndrome: a meta-analysis of reported symptoms. *Int J Epidemiol* 2005; 34: 1340-1345.

DeLong AK, Blossom B, Maloney EL, Phillips SE. Antibiotic retreatment of Lyme disease in patients with persistent symptoms: a biostatistical review of randomized, placebo-controlled, clinical trials. *Contemp Clin Trials* 2012; 33: 1132-1142.

Eikeland R, Mygland A, Herlofson K, Ljostad U. European

neuroborreliosis : quality of life 30 months after treatment. *Acta Neurol Scand* 2011; 124: 349-354.

Embers ME, Ramamoorthy R, Philipp MT. Survival strategies of Borrelia burgdorferi, the aetiologic agent of Lyme disease. *Microbes Infect* 2004; 6: 312-318.

Embers ME, Barthold SW, Borda JT, Bowers L, Doyle L, Hodzic E et al. Persistence of Borrelia burgdorferi in Rhesus macaques following antibiotic treatment of disseminated infection. *PLoS ONE* 2012; 7: e29914. Erratum: *PLoS ONE* 2012; 7. doi: 10.1371

Fallon BA, Keilp JG, Cordera KM, Petkova E, Britton CB, Dwyer E, et al. A randomized, placebo-controlled trial of repeated IV antibiotic therapy for Lyme encephalopathy. *Neurology*. 2008; 70: 992-1003

Fallon BA, Lipkin RB, Corbera KM, Yu S, Nobler MS, Keilp JG, Petkova E, Lisanby SH, Moeller JR, Slavov I, Van Heertum R, Mensh BD, Sackeim HA. Regional cerebral blood flow and metabolic rate in persistent Lyme encephalopathy. *Arch Gen Psychiatry* 2009; 66: 554-563.

Feng J, Weitner M, Shi W, Zhang S, Zhang Y. Eradication of Biofilm-Like Microcolony Structures of Borrelia burgdorferi by Daunomycin and Daptomycin but not Mitomycin C in Combination with Doxycycline and Cefuroxime. *Front Microbiol* 2016; 7: 62. doi:10.3389/fmicb.2016.00062

Garg K., Meriläinen L, Franz O, Pirttinen H, Quevedo-Diaz M, Croucher S, Gilbert L. Evaluating polymicrobial immune responses in patients suffering from tick-borne diseases. *Scientific Reports* 2018; 8(1). http://doi.org/10.1038/s41598-018-34393-9

Guyatt GH, Oxman AD, Vist GE et al. GRADE: an emerging consensus on rating quality of evidence and strength of recommendations. *BMJ* 2008; 336 : 924-926.

Haupl T, Hahn G, Rittig M et al. Persistence of Borrelia burgdorferi in ligamentous tissue from a patient with chronic Lyme borreliosis. *Arthritis Rheum* 1993; 36: 1621-1626.

Hodzic E, Feng S, Holden K, Freet KJ, Barthold SW. Persistence of Borrelia burgdorferi following antibiotic treatment in mice. *Antimicrob Agents Chemother* 2008; 52: 1728-1736.

Horowitz RI, Freeman PR. The Use of Dapsone as a Novel "Persister" Drug in the Treatment of Chronic Lyme Disease/Post Treatment Lyme Disease Syndrome. *J Clin Exp Dermatol Res* 2016; 7: 345. doi:10.4172/2155-9554.1000345

Hunfeld KP, Ruzic-Sabljic E, Norris DE, Kraiczy P, Strle F. In vitro susceptibility testing of Borrelia burgdorferi sensu lato isolates cultured from patients with erythema migrans before and after antimicrobial chemotherapy. *Antimicrob Agents Chemother* 2005; 49: 1294-1301.

Johnson L, Aylward A, Stricker RB. Healthcare access and burden of care for patients with Lyme disease: A large United States survey. *Health Policy* 2011; 102(1): 64-71. (www.healthpolicyjrnl.com)

Klempner MS, Hu LT, Evans J, Schmid CH, Johnson GM, Trevino RP, Norton D, Levy L, Wall D, McCall J, Kosinski M, Weinstein A. Two controlled trials of antibiotic treatment in patients with persistent symptoms and a history of Lyme disease. *N Engl J Med* 2001; 345: 85-92.

Krishnaveni M. A review on transfer factor an immune modulator. *Drug Invention Today* 2013; 5(2): 153-156.

Lawrence C, Lipton RB, Lowy FD, Coyle PK. Seronegative chronic relapsing neuroborreliosis. *Eur Neurol* 1995; 35: 113-117.

Lee DJ, Vielmeyer O. Analysis of overall level of evidence behind Infectious Diseases Society of America practice guidelines. *Arch Intern Med.* 2011; 171: 18-22

Lee SH, Vigliotti JS, Vigliotti VS, Jones W, Shearer DM. Detection of Borreliae in archived sera from patients with clinically suspect Lyme disease. *Int J Mol Sci* 2014; 15: 4284-4298.

Lewis K. Persister cells, dormancy and infectious disease. *Nature* 2007; 5(1): 48-56. doi: 10.1038/nrmicro1557

Meriläinen L, Herranen A, Schwarzbach A, Gilbert L. Morphological and biochemical features of Borrelia burgdorferi pleomorphic forms. *Microbiology* 2015; 161: 516-527.

National Guideline Clearinghouse. www.guideline.gov/summaries/summary/49320 (www.ahrq.gov/gam/index.html accessed 9 April 2019)

Pfister HW, Preac-Mursic V, Wilske B et al. Randomized comparison of ceftriaxone and cefotaxime in Lyme neuroborreliosis. *J Infect Dis* 1991; 163: 311-318.

Phillips SE, Mattman LH, Hulinska D, Moayad H. A proposal for the reliable culture of Borrelia burgdorferi from patients with chronic Lyme disease, even from those previously aggressively treated. *Infection* 1998; 26: 364-367.

Pillich H, Loose M, Zimmer KP, Chakraborty T. Diverse roles of endoplasmic reticulum stress sensors in bacterial infection. *Mol Cell Pediatr* 2016; 3(1): 9.

Preac-Mursic V, Pfister HW, Spiegel H, Burk R, Wilske B, Reinhardt S et al. Formation and cultivation of Borrelia burgdorferi spheroplast-L-form variants. *Infection* 1996; 24: 218-226.

Preac-Mursic V, Pfister HW, Spiegel et al. First isolation of Borrelia burgdorferi from an iris biopsy. *J Clin Neuroophthalmol 1993; 13: 155-161.*

Preac-Mursic V, Weber K, Pfister HW. Survival of Borrelia burgdorferi in antibiotically treated patients with Lyme borrreliosis. *Infection* 1989; 17: 355-359.

Schmidli J, Hunziker T, Moesli P, Schaad UB. Cultivation of Borrelia burgdorferi from joint fluid three months after treatment of facial palsy due to Lyme borreliosis. *J Infect Dis* 1988; 158: 905-906.

Shadick NA, Phillips CB, Logigian EL et al. The long-term clinical outcomes of Lyme disease. A population-based retrospective cohort study. *Ann Intern Med* 1994; 121: 905-908.

Sharma B, Brown AV, Matluck NE, Hu LT, Lewis K. Borrelia burgdorferi, the causative agent of Lyme disease, forms drug-tolerant persister cells. *Antimicrob Agents Chemother* 2015; 59, 4616-24.

Skogman BH, Glimaker K, Nordwall M et al. Long-term clinical outcome after Lyme neuroborreliosis in childhood. *Pediatrics* 2012; 130: 262-269.

Straubinger RK, Summers BA, Chang YF, Appel MJ. Persistence of Borrelia burgdorferi in experimentally infected dogs after antibiotic treatment. *J Clin Microbiol* 1997; 35: 111-116.

Stricker RB. Counterpoint: long term antibiotic therapy improves persistent symptoms associated with Lyme disease. *Clin Infect Dis* 2007; 45: 149-157.

Zhang Y. Persisters, persistent infections and the yin-yang model. *Antimicrob Drug Resist* 2013; 3. Doi : 10.1038/emi.2014.3

Ziska MH, Donta ST, Demarest FC. Physician preferences in the diagnosis and treatment of Lyme disease in the United States. *Infection* 1996 ; 24: 182-186.

Notes and observations pertaining to the 'fact finding' interview conducted by the Department of Health

I have been 42 years in the practice of medicine, and 25 of those years I have spent treating complex multi-systemic 'tick-associated disease' states. This often includes understanding the combined specialties of infectious disease, endocrinology, psychiatry, internal medicine, neurology, cardiology and rheumatology.

Five years ago the Department of Health and Human Services of New York State investigated my practice for the treatment of Lyme disease. After two years of appearing before the medical board to discuss 12 patients who had not registered a single complaint against me, I was charged with medical 'misconduct'. I was ordered to be 'monitored' for a period of three years. This was my response to the board:

1. Tick-associated illness is often misdiagnosed as other diseases by competent physicians, or ruled out as the basis of the presenting problem because of inaccurate laboratory testing. Minimal antibiotic treatment can often evolve into a chronic, persistent, recurrent illness.
2. There is a striking disparity between insurance-backed IDSA guidelines (which have not been updated in four years, and therefore are not currently comprehensive) and the existence of chronic persistent recurrent or relapsing borreliosis. ILADS, on the other hand (an organization of which I was a founding member), has

updated guidelines which are based on published research and recognize the existence of complex tick-associated illnesses. This body of physicians recognizes extended treatment options, including IV, multiple oral antibiotic regimens and intramuscular injections.

3. Patients enter voluntarily into my practice. I do not advertise. I have a personal website only. Individuals are usually referred by other patients who had been treated successfully. The patient population is drawn from around the country. Patients are always informed of the different guidelines and choose to participate in a treatment program consistent with ILADS thinking.
4. Since there are presently two schools of thought as to the correct diagnostic treatment, I believe therefore, that for this fact-finding interview to be fair and impartial, there should be at least one representative from the ILADS medical community, licensed in New York State, present in order to ascertain my competency in diagnosis, therapeutic decision making, treatment assignment and outcome results.
5. To the best of my knowledge, (including the selected cases under discussion), no formal patient complaint has been reported against me, here in the State of New York other than the prior case at our first meeting. Therefore, since I began treating patients here in New York City (an average of 300 new patients a year totaling 2100), formal complaints against me to the Department of Health have been non-existent. For that reason, I have not hired legal counsel.
6. A word concerning 'physical examination' of my patients: Since my specialty training is in psychiatry and family systems medicine, my interview and examination model has been derived from the psychiatric experience. Initially new patients are given one to two hours for work-up. Often, their histories are long, complicated

and accompanied by extensive medical records which require time before and after the session to review. Almost all patients have family physicians who have physically examined them many times. They have also seen multiple specialists who have examined them and recommended innumerable procedures (MRIs, extensive blood work, EMGs, sleep studies, EEGs, physical therapy, endoscopic exams, immune panels etc.). When needed I will exam the patient for a particular set of symptoms (auscultate for palpitations, shortness of breath; palpation for costochondritis or trigger points; exposure for angiomata and stria rashes etc., short neurological (finger-nose, nystagmus)). However, most of the consultation time is devoted to understanding the subjective world of pain, cognitive and psychiatric dysfunction, emotional changes etc.

7. Monitoring for adverse effects of treatment is based on symptom presentation over the course of illness. In the case of IV antibiotic therapy, this requires weekly nursing visits plus weekly CBC with differential, a metabolic panel and other supportive blood work when necessary. Blood testing for oral antibiotic therapy mostly depends on the patient's evolving symptoms and general progress, as well as scheduled visits to their family practitioner.
8. It should be noted that in the case of borreliosis, lab testing for specific IgG/IgM, ELISA, and Western Blot are useful primarily to help with the initial diagnosis. Regular Western Blot testing for treatment prognosis is minimally useful. Patient progress is measured by clinical symptom improvement and improvement in their quality of life.
9. Cystic forms have been shown to exist as a morphological phase of the *Borrelia burgdorferi* spirochete. At a later date, in a less hostile host

environment (no antibiotics) they can regenerate into a new generation of spirochete motile forms. The existence of these cysts limits current IDSA guidelines. Cysts appear not to be susceptible to the antibiotics used in the treatment of Borrelia; instead Flagyl, Plaquenil or Tindamax have been shown to be effective.

10. Although the physician representing the Department of Health has stated that he conducts the fact-finding interview in a 'fair and impartial manner' so that my competency may be judged, nonetheless his approach as represented by his 'line of questioning when applied to my records, is limited and misleading. In fact, it is apparent to me that his 'fact collection' has severely prejudiced my work. It creates a false understanding of my treatment of each patient and the outcome.

Practically all cases which have been chosen by the department for review have ended in a successful result. Their complicated multi-system problems for the most part improved. The patients whose charts were selected for review, returned to a 'healthier' quality of life. It should be noted that many of the cases under review had an average of six, sometimes up to 12 prior physician visits, with complete work-ups. Patients in spite of the specialists' input and treatments contacted me because they did experience sufficient relief from their symptoms.

Additionally, none of the cases chosen for the Department's review showed life-threatening or serious side effects from the treatments administered (mainly antibiotics alone or in combination). To the best of my knowledge, no patient registered a formal complaint with the Department of Health against me for any type of misconduct related to the treatment.

There have been no reported instances of fraudulent use of my medical license, including the use of unapproved or unnecessary testing procedures. There have been no reported instances of insurance fraud, excessive price gorging or fraudulent insurance reporting or charges for procedures that had never been performed. There are no reported instances of referrals to a diagnostic facility from which I profit.

I was disturbed that during this interview, I was never asked to discuss my treatment rational for any patients nor to elaborate on the decision-making process I used to prescribe the appropriate treatment and use of medication for the individual patient. In fact, I was never asked to discuss the outcome of any patient's treatment or whether the patient had in fact recovered from their symptoms. In short, whether or not the treatment was a success and the patient had improved.

No patient was ever contacted by the Department to discuss the quality of care they received at my hand, nor the ultimate success of the treatment, nor my personal medical conduct. Finally, it seems rather that a number of other physicians here in New York State known for their specific treatment of TBD have been summoned to defend their practice before the Department of Health.

It is ironic that New York State continues to be at the epicenter of this debilitating complex disease, and knowledgeable physicians rather than being positively cited for their time, energy and efforts on behalf of their patients, are instead being called to defend themselves against the charge of 'medical misconduct'.

Neuropsychological evaluation of a patient with tick-borne disease

Dr Leo Shea, Psychologist, President ILADS

'I was a prized executive by day and a super mom and wife at night and weekends. Now, that all has been lost to this illness. You can't imagine how devastating it is to have to rely on other people to organize your life and keep you and your loved ones functioning. I am so tired all the time and my brain is in a fog. I get exhausted and can't continue.'

This is a quote from a 46-year-old woman who had been diagnosed two years earlier with chronic fatigue syndrome and fibromyalgia. She was referred to me for a neuropsychological evaluation to determine her current level of neuropsychological functioning and assess her ability to meet job-related responsibilities.

Talking through her medical history, she said that in 2013 during a business flight to London she had developed sharp chest pains and difficulty breathing. She was seen in the Emergency Department at a London hospital and discharged. She was diagnosed with chronic fatigue syndrome and fibromyalgia. However, it had been two years with no improvement. And she had seen more than 10 medical specialists to date. It had been determined after two years that she had Lyme disease and Babesia.

At the clinical interview, she reported that her daily functioning had severely diminished. She had an overwhelming sense of malaise with exhausting fatigue that required a minimum of 10 to 14 hours of fitful sleep daily. She experienced constant and rotating bouts of pain and extreme weakness in her chest, neck, joints, rib cage, back, hips, hands, thighs and knees. She reported hypersensitivities to light and sound and cognitive reductions in attention, concentration, processing speed, short-term memory, planning and organization and multi-tasking.

Emotionally, she reported that she was moody, intermittently anxious, quicker to anger and prone to sadness over the reduction in her physical and cognitive abilities which, at times, occasioned notable depression.

Her academic and work history was impressive, having attended prestigious academic institutions of higher learning in Cambridge, Massachusetts and London, England. She had participated in university sports and was a ranked tennis player. She had exercised three to four times weekly prior to her illness. 'Now I do only minimal stretching/slow walking once a week, if it's a great week.'

Based on her perceived decline, she underwent neuropsychological testing to ascertain the impact of her Lyme disease on her intellectual functioning and her ability to carry out the responsibilities of her senior executive position. She was neatly dressed and groomed but her complexion was pale and when asked about her physical state, she replied that she was tired but, 'I'm learning to live with it. It's not fun but it's a part of who I am since I got Lyme. I used to be so organized I could multi-task like crazy but now I can't even get the children organized in the morning. It's very frustrating.'

She provided feedback on her first session of neuropsychological testing stating that at the end of that session she was exhausted. 'It's as if my brain exhausted my body. I got home and was barely able to do anything. I actually went to bed almost immediately.' During the second session she conducted herself much as she had during the first session, with dedication to the task but requiring periodic nourishment and stretching breaks.

She returned for her final session approximately two weeks later due both to a decline in her physical status characterized by general malaise and fatigue as well as having to attend to several family matters, all which took more time than she had expected..

Given her lack of effectiveness and efficiency in small matters, one could expect even greater problems were she to attempt a return to executive life with its demanding deadlines and where multi-tasking was an integral part of daily activities.

In summary, this 46-year-old woman ultimately was diagnosed with Lyme disease and Babesia after seeing more than 10 medical specialists at major medical insinuations in the US and UK. Neurocognitive weakness and compromised functioning were documented across a wide range of cognitive domains and confirmed that she was not able to access her innate abilities on a consistent basis due to the multiple physical symptoms and the cognitive reductions which compromised her functioning. Furthermore, her variability in performance limited her ability to access her strengths depending upon her state of cognitive fatigue or pain.

The results of her neuropsychological evaluation, with its frank cognitive deficits, variability and inconsistent application of cognitive strengths as well as her inability to maintain a consistent work effort over an extended period, confirmed the disabling effects of Lyme. This clearly was a major disappointment for this patient who had worked so diligently to achieve success both in her academic and business careers and in her spousal and family life.

While this is only one example of a Lyme patient, there are untold numbers of patients who are undiagnosed, misdiagnosed or under-treated, and who are suffering similar debilitating effects of this disease. It is important that when a person is diagnosed with Lyme or any other tick-borne illness that a neuropsychological baseline is administered as soon as possible so that targeted interventions can be delivered by the team giving treatment who are invested in the patient's recovery.

Tick-borne disease
Patient case histories

Dr Bernard D Raxlen

The following 10 case histories have been selected from my practice of more than 8000 patients to demonstrate the variability of the clinical presentation of the tick-borne disease syndrome. Unlike the six 'clinical intuitive narratives' used within the book to illustrate each individual patient's unique emotional space, these case histories are given as examples of what I and my fellow 'Lyme-literate' colleagues (LLMDs) deal with every day in our practices. They are, if you will, the 'dropped-through-the-cracks' patients referred to in this book – patients that LLMDs know only too well.

You will note that there are no discussions of individual treatment protocols for each patient case presented. Only the general category of the treatment used (intravenous (IV) or oral or intramuscular (IM)) and for how long a time. In each patient's case, their treatment included a specific supplement program. In IV antibiotic infusion treatments, those were supported by IV supplement therapy.

Case #1

A 34-year-old man came to my office complaining of headaches, weakness, stiff neck and fatigue. He had been experiencing increasing difficulty staying focused and had become very fatigued. He never felt rested, always feeling depressed with little or no energy. Earlier that year, he had become sound sensitive and so dizzy that he had passed out and gone into a seizure which put him in the hospital; this was dismissed as an anxiety attack.

The summer he came to see me, his migraines had become unbearable and he was experiencing total body weakness. An oval rash developed on his leg and hives started to cover his entire body. A series of scans and a spinal tap all came back negative; his only positive test was for Lyme.

He was treated with five days of IV Rocephin, and Doxycycline, which he stated helped make some improvement in his general symptoms. We ultimately went on to extend his IV antibiotic therapy, for up to 12 months.

Assessment: Chronic persistent borreliosis (Lyme disease) with neurocognitive involvement.

Case #2

A 43-year-old woman presented to our office with migrating joint pain, fatigue and memory problems. She reported problems with word retrieval, concentration, forgetting conversations with people, change in mood, easy irritability, feeling suddenly overwhelmed, drenching night sweats and a change in her temperament. These symptoms had been significant enough to affect her work. She could remember these symptoms starting approximately two years before, but they had recently worsened enough for her to seek treatment.

Her Western Blot test showed Lyme exposure on multiple bands (see page 27). We began treatment with oral antibiotic therapy, but did not see much improvement and switched to IV therapy for about six months.

Assessment: Neuroborreliosis and babesiosis.

Case #3

A 27-year-old woman cames to my office after experiencing multi-systemic symptoms with no apparent cause for the previous six months. These symptoms included: headaches, neck stiffness and tightness, joint pain, nausea, hot flashes, night sweats, photosensitivity, muscle weakness and soreness, decreased exercise tolerance, decreased energy, significant fatigue during the day, tremors in her hands, numbness and tingling in her back, and balance difficulties. In addition to these physical symptoms, she reported: trouble with her memory; difficulty thinking clearly; feeling confused: and being easily distracted.

Her Igenex Western Blot test came back positive for Lyme, even in accordance with CDC standards. Her Bartonella and Babesia titers were negative.

Assessment: Lyme disease.

Case #4

A 46-year-old wheelchair-bound woman came to the office with an extensive history of multiple sclerosis (MS). Ten years before, her knees had started becoming weak and she had had increasing problems moving her feet. She was soon diagnosed with primary progressive MS. Since that time she had become progressively worse to the point of no longer being able to walk. She had been prescribed several courses of steroids over the previous year, which she felt had made her much worse.

When she came to see me she was complaining of daily headaches behind her eyes and severe weakness in her arms. This weakness had started earlier that year, causing her to have difficulty holding her arms over her head, writing and completing fine motor tasks. She had significant neck pain, cracking and stiffness. She had continuous nausea and constipation, and needed to urinate every two hours. Her leg pain was a constant aching and stiffness; at times she was completely unable to bend her knees and her muscle would go into spasm. She experienced drenching night sweats and significant fatigue during the day. She was unable to sleep well at night due to the night sweats and her urinary frequency. Cognitively she was having trouble with word retrieval, clarity of thinking and memory.

Her blood tests come back positive for Lyme, Babesia, and Ehrlichia. IV antibiotic therapy was prescribed, for 12 months at minimum.

Assessment: Borreliosis, babesiosis, ehrlichiosis.

Case #5

A 45-year-old woman came to the office with an extensive history of multiple episodes of pneumonia and celiac sprue. She was complaining of heart palpitations, which caused both of her lungs to collapse, migrating pain in her right eye, right ring finger and the back of her neck. She suffered continual right-sided headaches which had become increasingly worse since the summer. Only a few months before she had had an episode of Bell's palsy, which caused drooling from the right side of her mouth and her right eye to become droopy. On any day she could have pain in any joint, burning in the bottoms of her feet and lower leg pain which would wake her from sleep. She had developed tremors and weakness in her extremities and found herself falling often when walking. Her sleep had become much worse, taking her one to two hours to fall asleep and then waking with night sweats and nightmares. Cognitively she found herself reversing tenses, word searching, increasing grammatical problems, forgetting the names of people she worked with, not being able to understand written text, and experiencing dyslexia-type reversals with words and numbers.

She had been bitten several times by ticks as a child, with multiple bull's eye rashes, but was never treated for Lyme disease. Over the last year, she had been prescribed tetracycline several times which she recalled helped the fevers subside and helped her start thinking more clearly. At the time of her first visit to my office, she had been on a course of Doxycycline.

After a positive Lyme test, we decide to continue the Doxycycline orally, ultimately adding IV antibiotic therapy for nine months.

Assessment: Chronic persistent neuroborreliosis.

Case #6

A 36-year-old woman came to the office with a four-year history of Lyme disease. She had experienced arthritic pain and swelling in her hands, and, after a positive blood test, was treated with Amoxicillin and Doxycycline for three weeks. This caused a severe Herxheimer reaction so she stopped the medication. Since then, she has reported being bed-ridden and unable to walk in addition to increasing problems with memory and disorientation. She has also experienced a 23 to 27 kilo (50-60 pound) weight gain.

She was a veterinarian and was constantly around animals, especially horses. Though her PCR blood tests were negative, her clinical symptoms allowed me to make a Lyme diagnosis. We started with oral antibiotic therapy and changed to IV antibiotic infusion for nine months.

Assessment: Chronic persistent neuroborreliosis.

Case #7

A 43-year-old, previously healthy man came to our office with a history of a tick bite two years before, and another one year later on his right thigh. Over the ensuing year, he had developed difficulty with his speech (slurring) and weakness. He had had an MRI which was negative. Since then he had had increasing symptoms, including trouble swallowing, shoulder pain (which he had injected with cortisone), testicular pain, problems blowing his nose because he was unable to take in enough air, and a general onset of fatigue. He was evaluated by an ENT specialist, a neurologist, had a stress test, echocardiogram, swallowing study, and dental examination which were all inconclusive. He said he did not have any headaches or vision changes. He had been experiencing difficulty falling and staying asleep, and had been having migrating joint pain.

Assessment: Borreliosis.

Case #8

A 10-year-old boy presented complaining of 'bugs crawling all over my body'. He had developed an increasing fear of separating on death. He had had a sudden attack of this in February when he had become more and more afraid. As the week progressed, he felt that he was going to disappear, his room was going to catch fire, and he felt the ground was going to fall beneath him. He refused to be touched and kept describing the sensation of bugs crawling all over him. He saw a psych pharmacologist and was also hospitalized because of the sudden changes. All testing at the hospital came back normal.

In my office, I conducted an Igenex Western Blot test that showed multiple band exposure. He was treated with oral antibiotic therapy for 12-16 months and all symptoms improved.

Assessment: Borreliosis.

Case #9

A 30-year-old man presented with a history of an atypical Lyme rash covering his entire body, especially his legs and lower back. He had been experiencing increasing exhaustion and decreased energy. In addition, he reported feeling 'less sharp' with memory and cognitive functioning. He had also suddenly developed seizures for which he was taking Depakote to control their activity.

Multiple Western Blot tests from different labs showed positive Lyme exposure. He also tested positive for parasite exposure. He was treated with a combination of oral and IV antibiotic therapy for 12 weeks.

Assessment: Borreliosis with co-infection.

Case #10

A 54-year-old woman, a registered nurse, was first seen in our practice almost a year before her next visit. That winter, she began to experience persistent pain and weakness in her arms. When she came back to our office, her symptom list now included back pain, with sore hips all the time, muscle tremors, hypophonia (soft speech) and fatigue.

She had a neurological consultation with Dr M, who diagnosed her early Parkinson's disease, affecting her right hand. He suggested the medicine Sinemet, but she declined it at that time. Seeking a second opinion, she saw Dr S, a cardiologist, who suggested an alternative diagnosis: neurological Lyme disease. Dr S recommended that she make an appointment with Dr P, a neurologist in Florida. The patient traveled to Florida to see Dr P, who confirmed the diagnosis and recommended antibiotic treatment, preferably intravenously. This was what brought her back to my office.

After running a series of tests and brain scans, she tested positive for Lyme disease on the Western Blot. Her brain scan revealed decreased blood supply in the high posterior parietal region of the brain. This allowed me to confirm the diagnosis of 'atypical, neurological borreliosis' presenting as Parkinson's disease.

Assessment: Neuroborreliosis presenting as Parkinson's disease.

Abbreviations explained

ADD	attention-deficit disorder
ADHD	attention-deficit hyperactivity disorder
AHILG	Ad Hoc International Lyme Group
AIDS	auto-immune deficiency syndrome
AIMS	Academy for Integrated Medical Studies
ALS	amyotrophic lateral sclerosis
AONM	Academy of Nutritional Medicine
Bb	*Borrelia burgdorferi*
BIA	British Infection Association
CACLD	Clinical Advisory Committee on Lyme disease
CAT	computerized axial tomography
CBC	complete blood count
CD4	glycoprotein found on the surface of immune cells
CDC	Centers for Disease Control and Prevention
CDNA	complementary DNA
CIPs	circuit impulse patterns
CLD	chronic Lyme disease
CLIA	Clinical Laboratory Improvement Amendments
CMIT	Collège des Universitaires de Maladies Infectieuses et Tropicales
CMV	cytomegalovirus
CNS	central nervous system (brain and spinal cord)
CSD	cat-scratch disease
CSF	cerebrospinal fluid
CWD	chronic wasting disease
DAkkS	Deutsche Akkreditierungsstelle, the ISO accrediting body in Germany
DNA	deoxyribonucleic acid
DSCATT	debilitating symptom complexes attributed to ticks
EBV	Epstein-Barr virus
ECDC	European Centre for Disease Prevention and Control
EEG	electroencephalogram
EIA	environmental impact assessment

Abbreviations explained

ELISA enzyme-linked immunosorbent assay
EM rash erythema multiforme ('bullseye')
ENT ear, nose & throat
EMECs electro-mechanical, electronical and computer science engineering
EMG electromyography
ESCMID European Society of Clinical Microbiology and Infectious Diseases
ESGBOR ESCMID study group for Lyme borreliosis
EUCALB European Union Concerted Action on Lyme Borreliosis
FFMVT French Federation Against Vector Diseases
FM fibromyalgia
fMRI functional magnetic resonance imaging
FUO fever of unknown origin
GAD generalized anxiety disorder
GI gastrointestinal
GP general practitioner
GPC Guias de Practica Clinica, Mexico
GPS global positioning system
GRADE grading of recommendations assessment, development and evaluation (method of assessing the certainty of evidence)
HAS Haute Autorité de Santé, France
HCSP Health Care Savings Plan
HHV6 human herpes virus 6
HPA Health Protection Agency (UK)
HPSC House Permanent Select Committee
ICD11 International Classification of Diseases 11th Revision
IDS infectious disease specialist
IDSA Infectious Diseases Society of America
IFA indirect fluorescent antibody
IgG immunoglobulin G
IGG same as above
IgM immunoglobulins of high molecular weight
IGM Same as above
ILADS International Lyme and Associated Diseases Society
INSERM French Institute of Health and Medical Research
ISO International Standards Organization
ITP idiopathic thrombocytopenic purpura
IV intravenous
IVIG intravenous immune globulin
KMF Comorian Franc (ISO currency code)
LB Lyme borreliosis
LD Lyme disease
LDA Lyme Disease Association
LLMD Lyme-literate doctor
LTT lymphocyte transformation tests (e.g. ELISpot-LTT)

MIN minimally invasive neurosurgery
MPFC medial prefrontal cortex
mRNA messenger RNA (ribonucleic acid)
MRI magnetic resonance imaging
MS multiple sclerosis
MUPS medically unexplained physical symptoms
NGC National Guideline Clearinghouse
NICE National Institute for Health and Care Excellence, UK
NIH National Institutes of Health, US
NHMRC National Health and Medical Research Council, UK
NHS National Health Service, UK
NLD not Lyme disease
NYC New York City
NYU New York University
OCD obsessive compulsive disorder
PANDAS pediatric autoimmune neuropsychiatric disorders associated with streptococcal infections
PCR polymerase chain reaction
PET positron emission tomography (an imaging technique that looks at function)
PHE Public Health England, UK
PHL Public Health Lab, Canada
PICC peripherally inserted central catheter
PLDS post-Lyme disease syndrome
POTS postural orthostatic tachycardia syndrome
PTLDS post-treatment Lyme disease syndrome
PTLS post-treatment Lyme syndrome
PTSD post-traumatic stress disorder
RMSF Rocky Mountain spotted fever
RNA ribonucleic acid
SPECT single-photon emission computerized tomography (3-D functional imaging)
SPILF Société de Pathologie Infectieuse de Langue Française, France
SSRI selective serotonin reuptake inhibitor (type of antidepressant)
STD sexually transmitted disease
STS Suffering the Silence
T1 type 1
T2 type 2
TBD tick-borne disease
TNF tumor necrosis factor (a cell signaling protein)
UKAS United Kingdom Accreditation Service
UN United Nations
UTI urinary tract infection
VEGF vascular endothelial growth factor
WHO World Health Organization

Index

Index